A COMPLETE Diet GUIDE FOR WOMEN

Dietitian Shreya

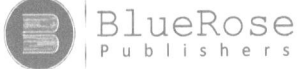

© **Dietitian Shreya 2020**

All rights reserved

All rights reserved by author. No part of this publication may be reproduced, stored in a retrieval system or transmitted in any form or by any means, electronic, mechanical, photocopying, recording or otherwise, without the prior permission of the author.

Although every precaution has been taken to verify the accuracy of the information contained herein, the author and publisher assume no responsibility for any errors or omissions. No liability is assumed for damages that may result from the use of information contained within.

First Published in September 2020

ISBN: 978-93-90396-83-2

sp@dietitianshreya.com
+91 8882 898 898

Cover Design:
Sukhpreet Singh

Typographic Design:
Ayushi Garg

Editor:
Dietitian Shreya

Distributed by: BlueRose, Amazon, Flipkart, Shopclues and available at our clinics too

About Dietitian Shreya (Author)

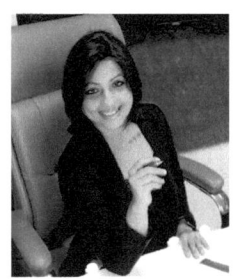

Dietitian Shreya is a Clinical Dietitian, Expert in Diabetes Management, Hormonal Imbalance and is also an Author/Freelance and Writer (Health & Lifestyle Nutrition).

Expertise in Diabetes Management, Weight Management and Hormonal Imbalance,

Post Graduate Diploma in Physiotherapy and Nutrition, Post Graduate Diploma in Nutrition and Dietetics.

Internship from PGIMER, gained experience working with FORTIS as a Clinical Nutritionist, also worked as a Dietitian for the Mid-Day Meal initiative (U. T. Education Dept.), and shared her valuable experiences as a TEDx Speaker.

Dietitian Shreya has been conferred with several awards and recognitions during her 14 years of serving as a dedicated Dietitian. She has been Given the Czar of North India title and the Lifestyle Journalist Women Achievers Award 2019. Lately, Dietitian Shreya was awarded Dainik Bhaskar Impact Awards 2019 for excellence in Diabetes Management and Hormone Imbalance by Mr. Anurag Singh Thakur [Minister of State for Finance and Corporate Affairs].

Subsequently, after the establishment of her diet clinics, Dietitian Shreya has been giving the best possible services to her clients. With her dedicated work, she is now the Director of Dietitian Shreya's Group. This includes:

20 Clinics Across India – At present, she has clinics in the Tricity, NCR-Delhi region, Gurugram, Mumbai, Lucknow, Jalandhar, Patiala, Kharar, Karnal, Ambala, Ludhiana and other regions of India. Going International soon.

DSA | Dietitian Shreya's Academy: Dietitian Shreya's Academy runs under her guidance to offer an internship of various durations to qualified Dietitians and Professionals.

AAHARIKA (N.G.O.): This is Dietitian Shreya's initiative under which, this organization takes care of the health of people from the underprivileged sections. They conduct health-promoting sessions, provide free education and healthy foods like gurchana, eggs, etc. to the community for making a small change in the world.

Heal Ayurveda Therapy: Dietitian Shreya's venture, the Heal Ayurveda Clinic in Phase 9, Mohali provides Panchakarma therapies for complete body rejuvenation and holistic health.

Trim-N-Tight (Slimming Beauty & More) Clinic: This is a clinic for giving easy and natural therapy sessions for individuals with cosmetic needs.

Online Dietitian Services: Dietitian Shreya is also providing her services worldwide and has a great team of expert Dietitians providing Mobile Dietitian services at patients' doorstep. It is for people who find it hard to visit the clinic due to impaired health or otherwise.

Staytox: Staytox is a lifetime experience with a quick gateway in the lap of Himalayan where you connect with nature and Ayurveda. It helps you to detoxify your body, mind and soul..Staytox helps in *achieving inner harmony with Naturopathy, Yoga and meditation sessions.The ultimate Detox Way & Stay to lose weight. At Staytox, we take a holistic approach to improve the health of our clients. Staytox venture started in November 2019.It was 3 days camp where people had achieved upto 3 kg weight loss. People from Mumbai, Lakhnaw, Delhi and other parts of the country had come to join this camp.They were given a warm welcome by our staff. The fresh air of the mountains and the serene atmosphere greeted them. Trekking, live cooking session, morning yoga and gardening were part of the program and people enjoyed all these activities. Staytox gave them so many unforgettable memories and an experience of a life time.*

Dietitian Shreya is an avid participant in public welfare activities. She frequently participates as a speaker and guides in health & wellness events for school kids and college-going students in various prestigious educational institutes of the region. Dietitian Shreya and her team organize health, wellness, and diet camps in corporate sectors also. She has also been a health counsellor for kids during their exams. Nearly 5 lakh people have connected and benefitted from the services of Dietitian Shreya's Group across the globe.

About This Book

Every day at my Clinic is a new learning and a new experience for me. Ranging from simple weight management to more serious cases pertaining to health issues like Diabetes, Multiple Sclerosis and even Tumor buildup, each day brings along with it so much more that I see, undergo and derive learnings from. This is not just a book, but is a first-hand account of all my experiences as a Dietitian and a Storyteller. In this book I shall take you through the true journey of a patient or a sufferer. We shall delve into the mindset of a patient, about how he/she faces the trauma of having a Disease, how they take up diets, and how in most of the cases, they defeat the Disease and live a life much healthier than ever before! Let's have a look at the Table of Content about the stories and the Diseases we are taking you through

Index

About Dietitian Shreya (Author) iii
About This Book vii
Prologue 1
My Women 4
Susceptibility of A Woman 9
Multiple Sclerosis 11
    Amitjot, 24 Years 12
    Mallika, 32 Years 15

Fibromyalgia 18
    Poonam Mishra, 29 Years 19
    Mrs. Harpreet, 43 Years 22

Mood Disorder Or Condition 25
    Rekha Thakur, 32 Years 27

Psoriasis 32
    Mrs. Reena Sharma, 48 Years 33
    Rhea, 6 Years 34

Thalassemia 37
    Mridula, 19 Years 39
    Geetika, 32 Years 42

Diabetes ... 44
- Sara, 7 Years ... 48
- Ananya, 12 Years ... 50
- Preeti, 44 Years ... 52
- Mrs. Harjinder Kaur, 54 Years ... 54
- Anupama, 25 Years ... 56
- Kritika, 29 Years ... 58

Thyroid ... 60
- Aastha, 28 Years ... 63
- Mrs. Amarjyoti Tripathi, 45 Years ... 65
- Mohsin, 40 Years ... 66
- Kirti, 17 Years ... 67

Typhoid ... 70
- Aasha, 26 Years ... 70
- Riya, 31 Years ... 72

Chronic Obstructive Pulmonary Disease (COPD) ... 77
- Jaysee, 21 Years ... 77
- Sweta, 60 Years ... 79

Jaundice ... 81
- Adamaya, 23 Years ... 82
- Mrs. Asha, 49 Years ... 84

Fatty Liver ... 87
- Mansi, 24 Years ... 88
- Mrs. Manjot Kaur, 37 Years ... 90

Digestion Gerd & Ibs 93
    Mrs. Amandeep, 46 Years 94
    Ruchi, 24 Years 96

Obesity 98
    Dilraj, 32 Years 99
    Mrs. Amrit, 43 Years 100
    Aayushi, 24 Years 102

Celiac 105
    Harkirat, 14 Years 107
    Jyoti, 8 Years 109

Bones 112
    Mrs. Shashi, 61 Years 114
    Mrs. Jaya Thakur, 38 Years 115

Cancer 117
    Mrs. Harminder Kaur, 57 Years 121
    Mitali, 20 Years 124
    Ripple, 36 Years 127

Kidney 129
    Shweta; 23 Years 129
    Priyanka, 32 years 131

Polycystic Ovarian Disease 133
    Mrs. Payal Garg, 26 Years 133
    Pallavi, 20 Years 135

Endometriosis 137
    Shiney, 28 years 138
    Mrs. Pratibha, 33 years 139
    Anu, 28 years 141
    Mrs. Anjali, 35 years 142
    Mrs. Harpreet Kaur, 45 years 145
    Mrs. Diljit Kaur, 50 years 146

My Inspirations 148
This Is Just The Beginning 154
Acknowledgements 156

PROLOGUE

Once in school, someone asked me, "What is your plan for the future, Shreya?" I told them in my low voice that I want to be a magician (because magic was a new craze for me). As time went on, my career choices varied. One time I wanted to be a car rallyist and another time I wanted to be a mountaineer. But I never thought that I would like to be a Dietitian someday. I was very active during my school and college time. I was into drama, play, dance, painting, yoga, cycling, Car rallying, badminton and participated in various other activities. After seeing me this much into extra-curriculum, my father always inspired me to live life happily but my mother was stressed about my career. After all, you know how mothers are!

I was a free bird who didn't know how to be in one place for a long time. When I was in school, I found cooking and reading about Indian food very interesting. So, when I had to choose my career option, I took home science, nutrition and dietetics. I was going with the flow!

When I was in college, I loved to read facts about nutrition and food. The more I read, the more I went into the depth of science and food. That time I didn't exactly know how wonderful our food is; that it has all the abilities to treat our body on its own.

I started my career as a Dietitian and worked for long hours in the hospital. After getting married to Sukhpreet Singh, I started it on my own. I met tons of people in my career and came to know about thousands of health issues that people face in different stages of their life; a woman is more susceptible in getting a Disease or any health issue due to her giving nature.

I think that in every stage of life, women grow but at the stake of their health. Every new phase of life demands something and a woman gives her health in return. I remember my mother gave up on her physical health to deliver us, sacrificed her sleep to feed us, food for work, bones, and muscles for negligence in recovering from deficiencies and mental peace for solving family issues. I know that being a woman is a blessing because we are stronger than men. We have beautiful body curves, breasts to feed young ones, we can bring a new life to the world, have a soft heart which is filled with emotions but somewhere down the line, we are taking our health for granted. I have seen mentally broken women, handicapped ones, depressed women, Cancer patients, diabetic women and everyone had one thing in common, which was negligence for their health.

Don't take yourself for granted. Health is the most precious thing you have. It's not only about physical health but it's about your mental, emotional and psychological health too. From the days I started, with everyone's blessings, I have managed to help so many children, girls and women in different aspects and in 2020, I celebrated the 14th Anniversary of the clinic.

This book will show you that diet can do miracles. By having healthy meals anyone can be treated from any Disease. I was not a person who was as health-conscious as I am today but my life experiences made me realize that you are what you eat and what you eat is who you are. These things are also mentioned in ancient Indian traditions and Vedas. They say that you think according to the food you eat. More you have good healthy food; more you will have good thoughts. I am not a qualified writer but I deeply wanted to write this book for all the beautiful people out there. It is not a self-help book but it is a piece of advice about how we can take care of ourselves and our families and friends. This book is for every man out there who wants his grandmother, mother, friend, sister, girlfriend, wife or daughter or any special one, healthy and enlightened. Let's gift my piece of advice to the most special person of your life and help her to not take herself for granted.

MY WOMEN

(A Story of My Mother)

"Shreya, come fast! Your breakfast is on the table. You will be late for school and I will be late for my office, hurry up!" My mother called me in the morning. I entered the room and found my favourite dish on the plate, gajar matar with parantha. I ran towards the food and said, "Genie, you are the best," with a big shiny smile. After having my breakfast, we both left for our respective places. She held my hand with one hand and her other hand was occupied with rolled breakfast. This was her daily routine. I found it tempting, that we can eat in this way and we need not care about a plate, table or chair. We can eat whenever we can or want.

My mother's appetite was very less, she never even told us about her favourite dish. Till now I don't have any idea about what she likes the most on her plate. Whenever I asked, she said, 'mujhe to sab kuch pasand hai' (I can have everything).

Being a working woman, she had shared everything of hers with us including her nutrition. We used to have aloo puri, aloo parantha on holiday but on her working days, we had easy to make food like poha, besan cheela, sheera, amaranth porridge etc. I was in a healthy environment since childhood in which my mother played a vital role. She is the reason that I am a Dietitian today. She was the one who chose this field for me by seeing my interest in Indian food and cooking.

She had time to feed us with vegetables, fruits, protein, rice, roti's, poha but didn't have the time to feed herself properly. I saw my mother compromised her nutrition and health for her family, husband, and kids. I saw her working 365 days in a year without a break. And now being a Dietitian, I don't want any mother to do it for anyone. Every mother gives unconditional love but they should not do it at the cost of their health and should take care of attaining proper nutrition for themselves. Every lesson that I learned from my mother has guided me to help many other mothers who have given up on themselves for their loved ones.

In case of my busy schedule, I always take care of my nutrition by adopting easy to cook food such as boiled eggs, salad juice, poha, porridge, amaranth ladoo etc. After marriage, I learned one more lesson from my mother-in-law: the importance of education. When Sukhpreet aka SP and I were busy settling our work, we used to be late in arriving home as we were busy opening our new branch in Ambala. At that time, my mother-in-law took great care of my daughter, Saadgi. One day my mother told me that she was feeling uneasy and having a mild headache, so I asked her to have a good sleep because she had not slept properly for the last 15 days. The next evening when I reached home late, I called Vikas (my caretaker), asked him for a glass of water and enquired about Saadgi and my mother-in-law. He told me that both of them were sleeping in their rooms. I first went to Saadgi's room and found her sleeping soundly; after that, I went to my mother's room and as I entered the room, I noticed that she was lying on the bed in pain. I immediately called Vikas to get a glass of water and ran closer to her and asked her if she was okay and what had happened. She replied 'pain' but was not conscious. I panicked and called my husband explaining to him the whole situation and at the same time, I asked Vikas and Anmol to bring the car so that we could rush her to the hospital. On the way, I called her doctor and explained to him the whole situation. He said that it was probably a heart attack and that we need to rush her to the hospital. She already had a stunt and the doctor said we might have to add another one.

I panicked badly on seeing Muma in that situation and after listening to the doctor's words, I was shut. I thought that this is not possible, that was a strong intuition. I checked her blood pressure and pulse rate, it was normal; like it didn't show any kind of abnormality in her heart. However, I asked the doctor to do an ECG when we entered the hospital as I had already checked her BP and pulse rate. The ECG was normal and we were relieved. There wa s no need for any stunt after the ECG. The doctor said that we shouldn't take any risk because she is a heart patient and we should do some more tests as he thought that there is a need for a stunt. I denied to do that and asked to consult an Orthopaedic Doctor as I had noticed swelling in her neck and upper back when we had laid her in the car.

At that point, everyone in the family said let the doctor work, please. But I knew what I was doing so I met the Orthopaedic doctor. He told our family that the pain was because of cervical as she had a problem of cervical spondylosis. That was the reason that her upper back and neck were stiff and swollen, and this was also the reason for her uneasiness. He said she would be fine soon but also asked us not to forget to make her exercise. That day I thanked God again because due to a thoughtful mind, Mumma wasn't going through any surgery again. In the same way, I don't know or I can't even count how many people are going through surgeries, spending money which is not even necessary.

Before making any decision, we should go through the technicalities. I know this is easy to say that don't panic in that kind of situation but when the situation arrives, we can't imagine anything else except the person who is suffering. But we should keep ourselves calm so that we can help the sufferer. My education saved my mother-in-law from an invasive procedure as well as saved our money. We all should be aware of basic information about our health.

Before this incident involving my mother-in-law, I was in the guilt of not being a good mother. It was all related to motherhood and being a working woman.

When you enter your new life, things change. Society changes with their point of views, when you do work only then people appreciate the wealth you have but criticize the time you give to your family and when you are a working mother, the society judges the decisions you make for your family because for them, you are a self-centered or selfish person.

The same happened to me when Saadgi was born. Being a Dietitian, I knew that a baby needs a mother's milk but people pushed me to give her water too. I knew that methi and ajwain water helps a lot in the feed but people said, "No, you should have more of milk and pinnis."

During my first child Saadgi, everyone had their own opinions and suggestions that the mother's milk (My feed) will be less if I did not have milk in my diet or did not have Panjeeri or Desi Ghee. So as a mother to avoid guilt, I indulged myself in guilt eating like Desi Ghee Panjeeri and butter, full fat milk without realizing that mother's milk is directly proportionate to the amount of quality diet, water and other liquids.

Even after I had listened to what people had to say, they still didn't stop nagging me about my child and kept on finding faults. Like, her poop was green which was normal to me but people still had something to say to prove that there was something amiss in my feed.

I later realized that they were not the people who did that to Saadgi but it was me who let that happen. I was weak to listen to them.

When I got pregnant with my baby boy (Shaurya) after 7 years of having Saadgi, I was at the age when people said that pregnancy is not easy.

When Shaurya came home from the hospital, those same people came back in my life to guide me on how to ruin the body of a kid. But this time I was prepared with all my heart and brain. Whenever they said something, I just smiled in reply.

I took methi ajwain water during my lactation; I exclusively breastfed Shaurya for 6 months, even after weaning him off I preferred less of gluten, more of millets and rainbow of nutrition. This way I managed to take care of my body my Postpartum nutrition too. And this time, a Dietitian mother won.

This knowledge of diet, the right kind of food and education, helps to win the battle which you are battling for yourself or your people. These small things inspired me to reach maximum people so that they get enlightened and make their life healthy.

SUSCEPTIBILITY OF A WOMAN

From making a "Doll house" to managing "Own house""

A woman is a wonderful word and an amazing creation of God. A woman is the one who can bring a new life on this Earth. What a miracle, isn't it? A woman has proved to be an emotional but multitasking person; her sixth sense is more active and more powerful than a man. Her ability doesn't need any of this explanation. More beautiful this creation is, more complicated it is. It is complicated because of its anatomy. At every age, a woman's body behaves differently and is susceptible to different Diseases or problems.

When a girl starts her life as a teenager, she experiences hormonal changes first. This teenager faces board exams, insecurity of looks, career options, first someone special and menarche. She grows physically, emotionally, psychologically, from school to college, knocked by puberty and new friends. When menarche hits her first time, it looks horrible (telling you by my own experience).

That intolerable pain, I can still sense it. It's the most beautiful and unbearable feeling altogether. Some start with normal periods and some with immense pain and irregularity. This can be possibly due to lower Haemoglobin, PCOD/ PCOS, fibroids, endometriosis and/or lack of nutrition in the body.

When a girl enters the phase of adulthood, all things change. Adulthood—it's such a wonderful chapter of life when a sense of responsibility comes. New dreams and hopes in one's eyes, with work stress and sleepless nights. In making the dreams come true, many women get knocked down by migraine, insomnia, Diabetes, cervical, asthma/COPD, UTI, ovarian Cancer, relationship problems, and depression.

Life goes on with the job and family of new people. A new life starts with the love of her life when motherhood hits. But conceiving is also not easy sometimes, good egg quality is important for that and the womb should be healthy to carry a baby in it. After conceiving, Anaemia, Gestational Diabetes, Thyroid, Oedema, morning sickness hold her hand. After baby, weight gain is normal and depression is also a part of life. Sleepless nights make woman vulnerable to anger and mood swings. Throughout her life, she faces dropped muscles, weak bones, low Immunity, Cancer, Multiple Sclerosis, Fibromyalgia, etc.

As she ages, she is even more susceptible to Osteoporosis, Breast Cancer, Muscle pain and lack of Synovial fluid. She is the one on whom our families depend completely. She can take care of everyone she loves but not of herself. Therefore, women out there, educate yourself for self and family, for having a good, healthy life with good nutrition. Once I read somewhere that "investing in Girls' education is the very best thing we can do, not just for our daughters and granddaughters, but for their families, communities and countries."

MULTIPLE SCLEROSIS

Before going through the stories of the people who went through this, let's have a detailed overview about the disease Multiple Sclerosis

INTRODUCTION

As the name suggests, Multiple Sclerosis (MS) — many lesions develop on parts of the brain and spinal cord. In this Disease, the insulated covering of nerve cells of the brain and spinal cord are damaged. Due to this damage, the ability of communication between the central nervous system (CNS) and other body parts disrupts. This disruption causes physical, psychological and sometimes, psychiatric problems. It is a common autoimmune Disorder affecting CNS. People among the age group of 20-50 are major sufferers and it is a long-term sickness.

CAUSES

- Destruction of the immune system
- Failure of myelin-producing cells
- Carry forward in genes
- Environmental factors
- Due to viral infection or infectious agents

SIGNS AND SYMPTOMS

- Fatigue and spasm
- Pain
- Muscle weakness
- Loss of sensitivity
- Blurred vision or double vision

- Difficulties with coordination and balance
- Problems with speech or swallowing
- Bladder and bowel difficulties
- Confusion, depression and unstable mood
- Worsening of symptoms due to exposure to higher than usual temperatures

DIAGNOSIS

- Blood tests
- Spinal tap (lumbar puncture)
- MRI
- Evoked potential tests

A PIECE OF ADVICE

- Gluten-free
- Lactose-free
- High protein diet
- Anti-inflammatory diet
- Science does not have any evidence that MS has any kind of treatment but in my experience, I have seen improvement in a few of my patients so don't lose hope.

IT WAS JUST AN ACCIDENT

Multiple Sclerosis

Amitjot, 24 years

"It all started in July 2018 with the accident of a student of masters who was living in a hostel at Panjab University, Chandigarh. One day, she was riding a scooter with her senior. Suddenly, an auto came in front of them and they had a bad crash and she got a deep head injury. People took them to the trauma centre, PGI. She was half-conscious and didn't understand what was happening around her. Her friends had arrived there and took her for an ultrasound and CT scan which was recommended by the doctors. Her senior was unconscious for 3 hours and had an injury on her feet. Her wound had bled a lot, and Amitjot's ear was bleeding too.

Her head was spinning. She vomited, slept and was awake at the same time. At 1 a.m when she opened her eyes, her mother and brother were in front of her and asked,"Putt kive aa tu? Tennu dard tan ne ho reya?" (How are you? Are you in pain?) she was not in a state to talk so she just blinked her eyes and closed them again.

The very next day, her parents took her back to Ferozepur, Punjab. When she recovered from the injury, she came back to the university to complete her research work, which was at the end of August 2018. She felt emotionally weak, was scared on the roads and felt a problem in turning her head. She was crying all the time in the hostel, probably because her friends had already left the place and she was alone there or may be, that accident left hidden scars on her mind. She thought that these were the side effects of the medicines which were given to her by the doctor. Her head pained every time she turned her head. She was feeling pain in her ear and her vision too was not clear.

She went to PGI and told everything to the doctor. He changed her medicine but the problem kept increasing. She went back to her home by the end of October after submitting her thesis. She told her parents about the problems she had faced in the previous months. So they took her back to PGI and spoke to the doctor. He said blood test and MRI is important, and that they should repeat it.

When they got the reports of her tests, the doctor told them that there were some serious issues in her brain. Her Myelin

Sheath had damaged her brain due to triggered autoimmune response of her body after the accident. But still, they didn't lose hope. After that, the doctor's voice did not reach her. Being a medical student, she knew that her life would be in a cage due to this. Her career and her dreams would be gone if the situation remained the same. The doctor was still telling something to her parents when she interrupted him and asked what will be the cure?

The Doctors told her that the medication would be strong enough to handle her weak body. Her body needed strength to start the treatment and with time, this problem would increase.

"I am here in front of you because my friend told me that you will help me to strengthen my body with nutrition. I need to get treated as soon as possible because I will go to the USA for my further studies in December 2019," she told me when she visited me for the first time. Her lips were trembling with fear but her eyes had a spark of hope in them.

I started her diet in February 2019. I gave her diets for strength and to boost up the treatment of MS. Right diet at the right point of time was important so I started with all gluten-free, lactose-free and more of anti- inflammatory diets.

It's December 2019 and she is already in the USA with the same spirit she wanted to be in. Her problem was at the initial stage so she got the chance to get her life back and this is all because of her will and the Law of Attraction. She is far better than before but she will carry forward the diet for her health.

"I wish her the strongest muscles and the strongest mind and a really great career that matches the high ambitions she had"

Lots of wishes and Love, Yours Truly, Dietitian Shreya!

THE BOND I SHARE WITH HER

MULTIPLE SCLEROSIS

Mallika, 32 years

A member of my Chandigarh team has a very smart personality and knows how to do her work efficiently. But from the last three weeks I noticed that her work was not efficient, she was making mistakes in those tasks which she was good at. I ignored for some time because I thought may be something had happened in her personal life and I shouldn't ask her directly. But when the situation went on the bad road, I called her directly to my cabin and asked her, "What happened? Why are you not doing your work properly?"

She said she has been off from some weeks because there was some problem in her life. She had a best friend name Mallika who lived in Canada, diagnosed with Multiple Sclerosis and the case was severe. Her grandmother was dealing with the same issue when she died in her later years but she is quite young to have this kind of problem in her life.

"When we were in school, we had a very good time. I used to talk to her a lot and share my emotional feelings, my secrets, my family issues with her. She is family to me. But after listening to her words about her health, I felt that someone had asked for my own heart. I love her and I didn't know that she is that important to me. We take our loved ones for granted because they are always there for us but when you get to know that maybe someday, they will not be there for you and will not listen to you anymore, will not react to your pointless talks, it feels like dying. I can't lose her. She is the only person I have on whom I can trust with my life. I can't lose her…" My team member lost her control and cried badly.

Her voice was shivering when she was telling her heart out. I hugged her and asked her to show me the reports. She said, "I know we could have helped her but her case is severe and doctors told her that there is no cure at this stage but her parents will try their best with immunosuppressants and some chemotherapy for her."

I asked to take a chance with her and said, "If you will not take a chance then surely you will spend your whole life in regret. If diet helped her to lift her medical procedure, then probably she would have been better right now. So, we will not interrupt her medicines but we will guide her to have some healthy diets which can help her to lift the medical treatment for her betterment."

I was convinced that if we do this the severity of this condition will be controlled. She talked to her friend and her family regarding the same and they were all in because they wanted to get her treated.

Her friend started having mood swings, blurred vision, and confusion regarding almost everything. She wasn't able to choose what clothes to wear, she wasn't able to call her mother on the phone because she forgot the password of her phone.

There were some precautions which I told them to take like don't make her feel that she is ill, don't let her know that she forgot something, the environment of the house should be very cheerful and positive which will bring some will power to her, have gluten-free diets, proper amount of salad and fruits, have an adequate amount of water, exercise to increase her concentration and focus. I asked her to start learning a new musical instrument or a new language, which will help to increase her brain activity.

They started all those things along with the medical treatment and after that, she was not depressed because she didn't know that she forgot something. Even my team member helped her a lot in this tough journey. And yes, we were right, her condition is not as severe as before and she is much better. She is still suffering from MS and we are all in it.

"Thanks to my teammate, who showed me the true meaning of Friendship and now I share the same bond with Mallika.

She even invited me over for her wedding and it is gestures like these that really move me and make me realize that I did manage to make a difference in people's lives and I stand grateful for that"

Lots of wishes and Love, Yours Truly, Dietitian Shreya!

FIBROMYALGIA

Before going through the stories of the people who suffered from this, let's talk about the disease Fibromyalgia.

INTRODUCTION

Fibromyalgia is known as a pain syndrome. It is characterized by chronic muscular pain. It includes fatigue, cognitive disturbance, mood Disorders, insomnia etc. In the morning, stiffness is very common in the body. Pain spreads to joints, tender points and central nervous system. However, it is related to some specific Diseases like infections, Diabetes, rheumatic pathologies, psychiatric or neurological Disorders etc.

Fibromyalgia is more common in women compared to men and it increases with age.

CAUSES

There is no specific cause of Fibromyalgia but it can be prompted by numerous physical or emotional stressors which include infections as well as trauma. Fibromyalgia is common in patients affected by autoimmune Disease.

SIGN AND SYMPTOMS

- Musculoskeletal pain – Initially in the neck and shoulders.
- Fatigue – Especially when waking up from sleep.
- Cognitive disturbances
- Anxiety
- Depression
- Migraine

- Gastroesophageal reflux Disease (GERD)
- Palpitations
- Disturbed Sleeping Pattern
- Psychiatric problems

DIAGNOSIS

- Diagnosis is complicated and often missed because the symptoms are indistinguishable or generalized

PIECE OF ADVICE

- Patient education
- Exercise
- High protein diet
- Gluten-free diet
- Lactose-free
- Hey women, you are very strong, don't let your Fibromyalgia dominate your muscles!

RAY OF LIGHT

FIBROMYALGIA

Poonam Mishra, 29 years

One day, Lakshman Ji received a phone call in the early hours of the clinic. Someone asked him about the address and said, "I want to meet Shreya." Lakshman Ji guided her to the clinic and told her that she needs to wait for a while because the meeting time will start after 30 mins. She refused to wait and said, "I just want to meet her now or you give me her number. I will call her." My staff told her that they had informed me and I was coming to meet her early.

As everyone told me already about what chaos she had created, I drew her in my mind. But when she entered my cabin, I couldn't recognize that she is the same person they have told me about because she was so calm, composed and smiling. I welcomed her warmly; we sat down on the sofa after shaking our hands and exchanging names. I began with a sorry for making her wait for me for so long. She said, "Oh! No-no- no… that's completely okay. I am the one who came early so no need to apologize." I was a bit confused but then blew up the thoughts and started our conversation. "So, tell me about yourself." She said, "I am Poonam Mishra and I am from Saharanpur but shifted to Chandigarh for a couple of months to my relatives (bua) to take a break from my routine. I am 27-28 years old and unmarried." She made a very confusing facial expression about her age. Her rational mood swing behaviour and confusing facial expression on her age had clicked some things in my mind but I didn't express it to her.

"I am facing very severe pain in the muscles and joints of my body; can you help me in this?" she asked. I said with a broad smile, "Yes, of course, you will be okay very soon." But she was unaware about the severity of the problem that I had sensed. For the complete diagnoses, I asked her some more questions. How is your sleeping pattern? Is it disturbed? Is there any stiffness you feel in your body in the morning? Do you have headache or hair fall? What about mood swings?

Some yeses and some noes I got from her. She said, Mujhe thik kar do aap mai dukhi ho chuki hu ab. It's like every time I wake up in the morning, I feel the same low, tiredness, and irritation. Sometimes I feel happy and sometimes I feel like crying out loud; multiple things cross my mind and I start crying. I feel so alone now. I don't have anyone to share all these things with. And what should I discuss? I am a person who is tired of body ache? People will laugh at me…"

I felt that pain she was feeling because she was, not even aware of what she was facing. She told me everything about her health and I suggested her more of proteins like eggs, quinoa and amaranth, and fragrance diffusers in her room, daily sunlight exposure to her body and her room. I asked her to visit and see me on every fourth day for the follow-ups so that I could know her problems minutely.

She visited me according to our discussion and I came to know that her medical parameters are capturing her mental state too. She used to forget so many things; she even forgot the conversation we had verbally. She remembered only those parts of the meeting which were written in her diary. That was a shaking moment for me. Because if during that period we did not control her symptoms of Fibromyalgia, then surely it will get worse. My team and I were very confident that we will handle her efficiently. Meetings with her had always been a task because, during every new meeting, we came to know a new fact about her that she had forgotten to tell us before. We prepared a diary for her and wrote every minute details of our meeting, which helped us loads.

She was improving satisfactorily, but after 3 months, she had to go back to her hometown, where she could not pursue the diet. I tried to call her on every fourth day to know how she was. But after a few weeks, my calls remained unreciprocated. I was discouraged and thought she was improving very well but our conventional society won't let people live liberally and blissfully. With time, I transformed my anger into a new fume and started normally.

Two months later, my team got a call from her. She wanted to talk to me. At first, I refused to talk to her because she had let me down but then I took her call with excitement.

"I am happy, very happy, just because of you, Shreya Ma'am. You helped me in that period when everyone misunderstood me. You were the ray of light for me. Thank you so much, ma'am, and yes, I am getting married so please do come here! I will send you an invitation. Are you listening? Hello...? Hello...? Are you there...?" she said.

"I am relieved that you are happy," I said and the sobbing sound was still there but this time, it was from my side.

For me this case is a perfect of the Law of Attraction.

Take away Tip: You will get whatever you want if you attract it with that burning desire.

Yours Truly, Dietitian Shreya

LONG JOURNEY TO COVER

FIBROMYALGIA

Mrs. Harpreet, 43 years

I remember months ago when we were planning to celebrate Holi, one of Diet counsellors got a phone call. Since it was an unknown number and we have a policy that we can't ignore any unknown number, she picked the call and spoke to the person walking out of the celebration. She came inside after 30 minutes when the meeting was over. She said, "Oh my bad! I missed the meeting." Everyone laughed at that and one of them said, "Yes, it's your bad that you missed it." She told us that she has a case to discuss with all of us. She looked puzzled but I said sure. She told us that there was a man on the phone, Mr. Harbans Singh. He came to know about us through a family member who watches our videos on YouTube. He said his wife, Harpreet, is suffering from Fibromyalgia from the past one year. They have been to every doctor they could go to but it hadn't been fruitful. Ten months ago, the doctor told him that she could be bedridden in a few months and that he should take care of her. In the starting, they were taking it very casually. Whenever she felt pain in her body, she used to take pain killers. As a result, she was now bedridden and sometimes she called them by their name and sometimes she did not even remember her own name. Her medicines were still going on but they were not helping her at all.

So, I asked him if we can meet. I said, "I know it's difficult for you but we can discuss the complete case with you. "He said, "My wife and I are alone here. Our children are in Australia and the maid is on holiday due to Holi. But I really want to see my Harpreet alive like before. Can you come to our place? If it's possible for you."

The case was critical and a medical urgency, so I said yes to him and told them that I'll meet them the next day, on the day of Holi itself.

She said all this albeit with a smile on her face, with nervousness and then was waiting for everyone's response. I was astounded by my team. From where was my team congregating this drive and compassion, that they could sacrifice their holidays or celebrations of life.

I said, "It's a perfect plan; we are going to their place and then celebrate Holi with pride."

The next day, I wished happy Holi to my family and friends, kissed my two small munchkins with colours and left them for an hour. When we were heading towards their place, I saw the different colours of Holi, life, humans and then thought of all that Mrs. Harpreet was missing and that thought brought tears in my eyes, but I wiped them off as soon as possible because I felt blessed that God had chosen me for this work.

We reached there. Mr. Harbans Singh, and called for his wife, was 58 years old who lived in a big house with his wife. His house was painted in pastel colours. After seeing his lifestyle, I found that yes, money is important but not more than health. What if you have lots of money but don't have a body on which you can spend it happily.

We went inside to meet Mrs. Harpreet; she was a beautiful lady aged 52 years. I saw her photographs on the wall. She was very lively. Her smile was bold, aloud and captivating. It was a real pain to see her as a different Harpreet on the bed. We saw all the reports and discussed everything with her husband. She was talking to us but she didn't remember much about her own story. Her Erythrocyte Sedimentation Rate (ESR) was very high. Deficiency of vitamins, lacking in iron, pre-Diabetes condition, memory loss, crying most of the time etc. were her symptoms. We planned the diet accordingly, which included eggs, quinoa, amaranth, pulses, soup, palak, gluten-free oats, ragi, jowar, bajra, supplements of vitamins, zero carbohydrates/lactose/gluten, steam bath, sunlight exposure in the morning, heat-producing food, sage tea etc.

For the next meeting, the diet counselor who had spoken to Mr. Harbans went there to meet them. I spoke on video call with her because I was not in the clinic as I was travelling for a Meet and Greet session in Mumbai. During the call, I found them to be more vibrant. Their house was welcoming sunlight and positivity. Although in fifteen days I couldn't make any drastic change, she talked more this time. She came back and told me that Harpreet Ji was improving. It has been 6 months of our journey and she is improving well. It took time to take every step but every obstruction was a challenge for us. And we all fought it with a smile. She can sit now, her memory is better, pain is less, and deficiencies are recovering now. There is a substantial journey to cover yet. Her story made me believe that the prayers of Karvachauth are not only from the women's' side but also it is from the men's side. I wish them years of togetherness and a healthy and joy filled life ahead!

With Respect, Yours Truly, Dietitian Shreya!

MOOD DISORDER OR CONDITION

Before I narrate to you a really special story, let's understand the emotions.

DEPRESSION

It is a severe mood Disorder. It can affect your feelings, thinking, sleeping and eating patterns or way of working. It can happen at any age. There are certain periods when this Disorder can overcome your mental health such as:

— Postpartum depression – mother experiences this after giving birth to her baby.
— Psychotic depression – one can hallucinate in this condition (depression with psychosis).
— Seasonal depression – the onset of depression during winter because of less sunlight.
— Bipolar Disorder – mood on extreme levels, high or low.
— Premenstrual Dysphoric Disorder (PMDD).

SIGNS AND SYMPTOMS

— Persistently sad and anxious
— Feelings of hopelessness, guilt or worthlessness
— Negativity
— Bad temper
— Loss of energy
— Feeling fidgety
— Difficulty in early-morning awakening or oversleeping
— Thoughts of death or suicide, or suicide attempts

RISK FACTORS

— Family history of depression
— Major life changes like trauma or stress
— Physical infirmity and medications

OBSESSIVE COMPULSIVE DISORDER (OCD)

OBSESSION: It is the repetition of thoughts, mental images that cause anxiety. Common symptoms include:

— Scared of germs or infection
— Violent thoughts for self or towards others
— Want things in an ideal order or perfect symmetry.

COMPULSIONS — it is a repetitive action in response to obsessive behaviour. Common compulsions contain:

— Unnecessary cleaning or hand wash
— Placing things in a particular order
— Frequent inspection of electric switches, doors, windows etc. to check if they are off and closed or not.

Obsessions or compulsions or both can interfere in life activities like in school, workspace, personal relationships or in a social gathering. Every person doesn't show the same symptom, they may have the OCD of checking on things twice or thrice. This kind of symptom or OCD can get worse with time. People start alcohol or drugs to calm themselves down or to not do this repetitive behaviour.

It can be due to one's family history, brain function, environment factor, or surroundings. PIECE OF ADVICE

— You need to be very strong and fight from depression
— Whatever thing is making you upset, you have to avoid it; even if that thing is your closed one, it's high time to say goodbye.

SURROUNDED BY FAMILY

DEPRESSION

Rekha Thakur, 32 years

"Hey… how are you doing? Looks like I am having a surprise visit from my client or I can say my extended ex healthy-family member," I told Rekha Thakur.

I was really happy to meet her again especially after such a long time. She had shifted to Canada three years ago, for her higher studies with the love of her life, her would-be husband. She came to me for her bridal preparation for skin and egg quality diets.

When we met again now, she was a grown-up woman. We sat on the black couches with the cushion on our lap and were feeling like friends getting together. We were talking about her life in Canada and everything but her happiness was missing. She was telling me that she was good there. Then she told me that she will be in India for 2 or 3 months probably. I asked her the reason to be here in India.

She said she came here one month ago for the cremation of her mother. Her life completely changed after the death of her mother because she took care of her from her childhood and being a single parent, she had done a lot for the family. Rekha was shattered completely. I told her that this is a phase that has to come in everybody's life. But your life is in front of you, so just keep good memories of her and look forward.

She said, "I wanted to start the diet again which can help me keep my mind calm. I want to relax and feel good." I started her diet for her good mental health like chamomile and sage tea, food with less oil, fruits and salad and moringa tea. After two months, she went back to Canada.

She called me after 6 months of our meeting and said, "I am not feeling well. I feel like I want to cry all the time. It's been one month and I am feeling like this only. I have been losing myself somewhere. I have never had this kind of irritating personality ever. I am not able to stay happy for long. Even if I feel happy, it doesn't stay for long. I don't want to get up in the morning and face the world; many times, I don't feel like coming home at night. I have no idea what this is. I am not sharing good relations with my husband also. It's like I have lost all senses. It has exaggerated after the death of a good friend of mine two months ago."

I got to know that she is in depression. I put her case online and on call, I was helping her. I planned her diet and tried to make her positive about her life. I told her to take natural light, be surrounded by loved ones, stay away from screens like laptops or mobiles, and find hobbies which could make her feel happy.

She started it and tried to talk to her husband about her condition too. He understood her mental health and helped her in every possible way. He took work from home so that he could spend more time with his family. She was feeling much better when she was talking to me on the phone. "It's not perfect but I am relieved that you, my family and my inner strength are helping me to come back.

Thank you so much for listening and understanding me and helping me like this," she said.

I was happy to hear her voice and by knowing the power of listening.

Take Away Tip: Depression can be clinical too so take it seriously. Also, if the depression is due to any sort of deficiencies like iron, Vitamin D, Vitamin B12, Ferritin or Hormonal Imbalance, then this silent disease can be well taken care of with few changes in Diet. So next time, try a cup of Chamomile Tea with a piece of chocolate and a warm hug and caring words with your loved ones!

Yours Chocolaty Friend, Truly, Dietitian Shreya!

LADY WITH THE TISSUE PAPERS IN HER BAG. FOR REMOVING MAKEUP OR FOR WIPING TEARS?

OBSESSIVE-COMPULSIVE DISORDER

Mrs. Paramjeet Kaur, 49 years

I was on holiday and at that time, I generally switch off my phone for some days. So, when I switched on my phone, I got a message from the clinic. It said that Mrs. Paramjeet Kaur was calling to get an appointment to meet me; she was coming from Delhi to Chandigarh just to meet me. She said that the meeting is urgent so she needed a date for the meeting. I replied that my flight will land in Delhi and if it's urgent, then fix my appointment with her at the Delhi clinic.

Mrs. Paramjeet was already our client who was taking a diet course from my online team. I remember when I was discussing her case with one of my staff members, she told me that the case is of weight loss only.

When I visited the clinic, I met so many people there. They were glad and surprised to see me. It's not that bad after a good holiday.

Mrs. Paramjeet had arrived and met me warmly. She said, "I was planning to meet you but sorry, I kept calling your staff for the appointment." I said it's okay and asked her about her progress although I had already seen her form which was maintained by my team. She had lost weight well in the start but then her form was filled with lots of cheating, skipped periods, couldn't sleep well, couldn't follow the diet and reached on the same number from where she started.

She showed her diary to me; it was wrapped in a tissue paper and she was picking it up like it was a dirty cloth. I asked her why she had wrapped it in a tissue paper. She said that it fell in the car so that was the reason to wrap it. Even before putting her elbows on the table, she pulled out the tissue from her handbag, cleaned the table and then put her elbow on the table. She said, "I am doing well, thank you. I am just not losing weight because I didn't have time to do it."

After watching her actions, I asked her how many people are there in her family. She said, "We are four —my husband, two children, and I. My daughter got married and has settled in the US, my son is in IIT Mumbai, and my husband stays on tour for his business. I was also a working woman but later, I chose to quit the job and stay at home."

"So, what do you do the whole day?"

"I read the newspaper, watch news or serials, prepare some good food for myself, cleaning and cleaning. I spend my maximum time in cleaning. It's so dirty, you know? Every corner of my house needs to be clean, clothes to be washed and then ironing of clothes; it's a tough job, you know. It demands perfection."

I figured out that she was alone from inside too. She had OCD (obsessive-compulsive Disorder) because of her loneliness. She was pretending that she was alright and happy in her life and daily routine but she was not. She wanted to clean everything and didn't want to see any crease on clothes because she wanted to see her life like that — no crease, no dirt. I asked her to make a call to her husband once so that I could speak to him. She asked, "Why do you want to talk to him? He must be busy somewhere. "But finally, she agreed to give her phone to me.

I asked Laxman Ji to take her for the quiz activity which was happening in the sitting area.

Meanwhile, I told everything to her husband and asked him to take care of her by all means. He didn't trust me completely but still, I asked him to spend some time with her.

I have changed her diet plan and increased the feel-good hormone diet. I gave her chocolates to eat if she felt low, fresh Aswagandha tea twice for her calmness, more of a Protein diet for her muscles and healthy Carbs and Fats for the mind.

I asked her about her hobbies and she told me that she loves to knit sweaters. I said, "In the next meeting, will you gift me a sweater for my daughter, Saadgi? She agreed and left. The journey continued for the next 6 months."

In the last meeting with her, she came to Chandigarh and gifted me a black hooded sweater for Saadgi and said thank you with an actual calm smile.

I replied, "I am happy that you are not carrying a tissue box anymore."

I wish every woman on this planet carries a tissue for her lipstick and not for some unworthy tears!

Your Buddy for life, Dietitian Shreya!

PSORIASIS

A SKIN DISEASE

It is an autoimmune skin Disease, in which the skin gets patches, scales and redness. These patches are generally around the elbow, palms, armpits, genitals (inverse psoriasis), back, scalp, swollen or painful joints (psoriatic arthritis) and knees or on the entire body (erythrodermic psoriasis). It can also affect the sole of feet, mouth (plaque psoriasis) and nails (nail psoriasis).

In psoriasis, the growth of skin cells is elevated; which forms extra skin on the body and it further forms patches and scales that can be itchy as well as painful. Treatment of psoriasis is to stop the growth of the skin cells. Changes in lifestyle, avoiding stress, quitting smoking can help to control the symptoms.

SIGN AND SYMPTOMS

- Red patches on the skin
- Scaling spots
- Cracked skin
- Itching or burning problem
- Swollen and stiff joints
- Makes performing routine tasks difficult

PIECE OF ADVICE

- Get the allergy panel test done, know your IgE levels;
- Don't apply anything on the skin without knowing the ingredients
- Have your own personalized diet plan made by a Clinical Dietitian.

BEAUTIFUL SKIN

PSORIASIS

Mrs. Reena Sharma, 48 years

When I joined my clinic after the delivery of Shaurya, it was like a rebirth for me. I was completely new again, full of energy, positivity and happiness. That day I came early to the clinic because I was so excited about that. After a morning meeting with my team, I started to meet clients who were waiting in the waiting area.

There was a face which was new to me. She was wearing a yellow suit with a black long coat and her face was glowing with a smile. When she entered the cabin, she greeted me with a smile and told me that I have made her wait for so long. She wanted to meet me fora long time but the circumstances and situations were at peak and we couldn't meet till that day. "I am Reena Sharma from Una, Himachal Pradesh" she started, "I have a skin issue from the past 5 years. It's prominent seasonally — painful in winters and itchy in summers." Her hands were full of scaly skin and her neck was also the same. She showed me her elbow too, it was full of red patches. "I have consulted with so many doctors, some had given me steroids while some gave an ointment to apply but it made my skin worse. My joints were swollen and painful after that. I am not comfortable to go on outings with my friends and family because people give me weird looks as if I am carrying some serious communicable Disease. Many times, I feel ashamed due to my condition. After tolerating this problem for 5 years, I am tired of consulting doctors and having allopathic medicines. My niece had suggested me your name as she took diet from you online for her pregnancy so she asked one of your team members regarding my issue. My niece got a positive response from your side and asked me to meet you only, so I have been trying from 2 months but today is the day when I could come."

"Yes, this problem can be controlled but you need to restrict the gluten in your diet and diet is not something like a magic stick, which can show results in a blink. Your condition is severe and it will take time to get treated, so you need to be patient for the treatment. It will work slowly and will take time because it's your elevated skin cell growth which could only come under control slowly," I told her everything in detail.

Her age was 48 years and her ageing were fast so the treatment could take its own time for recovery.

She agreed to wait as long as she could stay dedicated to diet as she had many food allergies which she had to avoid throughout life along with high protein, no raw food were the main points of her diet. She is still a part of our healthy family and got treated for her hands and elbow first. She is having her diet dedicatedly and now she is comfortable in her beautiful skin.

I hope this case study will inspire everyone to take care of the largest organ in our bodies "The Skin". Shade of the skin doesn't matter, the smile on your face does!

Truly yours, Dietitian Shreya

MATCHING HAIRBAND

Psoriasis Rhea, 6 years

My husband loves his relations and celebrates them by spending time with them. He has many friends and a few of them are very close to him. We share family-like relations with a few of our friends. One day, he and his friends planned a get together at our home. Rohit and Ekomjot, visited our house that night and spent a good time together in our fun area and also went for a gehri (roam around) in the city. They were talking about their lives and discussed some family things too. During these conversations, Rohit told SP about his Daughter, Rhea. She was having psoriasis. SP did not know too many technical terms, so he asked what exactly it is. He told SP, "Psoriasis is a skin Disease. Though it is at its early stage, it's increasing day-by-day. I can't see my daughter in pain and in that phase where she is scratching her body a lot. She is so young for all this — her age is just 6 years. Sneha, her mother, is also very worried and is searching for doctors or a possible way to treat this problem. The environment of our home is so different from the past one month since we came to know about the condition of Rhea. And today, this party is an escape from that environment for me. I feel so helpless when Rhea cries because of the itching on her skin."

"I will see what I can do for you. I know there will be a way out of this condition. I will talk to Shreya also regarding this." SP sympathized with Rohit.

When SP told me about his conversation with Rohit, I was so shocked because psoriasis shows different symptoms in different individuals. I called Sneha and asked her to come home with her daughter. I was also nervous because it was my first case of psoriasis. I made the call because I couldn't let Rhea bear that pain.

They came home and I met Rhea, she was looking like a doll. She wore a frock of brown colour with a matching hairband; her hair was so long. We sat on the swing in our balcony and discussed Rhea's skin. Sneha was also allergic to strong smell and dust, which made Rhea an atopic individual. I asked Sneha to take a break from her research on psoriasis and just take care of Rhea. We could undo the situation with healthy diet because it was at an early stage. "And I know you, you will never take her diet for granted. So, shall we start?" I said.

After a long pause, she agreed and said, "I will do it but I need positive results. I trust you, Shreya, so I am ready to take this risk. I hope you will not break it." I was nervous but sure and committed to doing my job. I started with her diet plan according to her school timings. I suggested Sneha to give her eggs, soup and say no to gluten also. She did exactly what I told her to do. Rhea's skin responded after 1.5 months and Sneha showed her first smile after so long.

October 26, 2019, there was a Diwali party at my home and SP invited our friends. I saw Rhea after so long. She was then 16 years old and looked just like Sneha in her features.

Take Away Tip: There is no age too early to start a correct Diet! Don't let the disease say," Here I Come, Ready or Not"

THALASSEMIA

Not so Bright

INTRODUCTION

Thalassemia is the most common genetic Disorder in which the formation of Haemoglobin (protein in red blood cells (RBCs) which carries oxygen) is abnormal or inadequate. This abnormality leads to Anaemia due to the destruction of a large number of RBCs and lowers the concentration of oxygen in all parts of the body. Lack of oxygen in the tissues and organs can cause pain in the body or increase laziness. Thalassemia is classified into two types depending on the severity of symptoms: thalassemia major (also known as Cooley's Anaemia) and thalassemia minor.

Thalassemia Major – It is known as Cooley's Anaemia and out of the two types, thalassemia major is more severe.

SIGNS AND SYMPTOMS

— Pale skin
— Poor appetite
— Failure to grow
— Irritability
— Spleen enlargement
— Anemia
— Growth retardation
— Jaundice
— Leg ulcers
— Skeletal changes resulting from the expansion of the bone marrow

- Wider bones, abnormal bone structure and increased risk of broken bones
- Slow growth rate; delayed puberty
- Heart Diseases; heart failure

CAUSES

- Genetically transferred
- Mutation in genes

TREATMENT

- Blood transfusion
- Iron chelating
- Supplements of iron-folic acid
- Bone marrow transplant
- Surgical removal for an enlarged spleen

Thalassemia Minor – Thalassemia minor is usually clinically asymptomatic but sometimes causes mild Anaemia. When both parents are carriers, there is a 25% risk at each pregnancy of having children with homozygous thalassemia.

SYMPTOMS

- Drowsiness
- Weakness
- Pale skin
- Facial bone deformities
- Retarded growth
- Abdominal swelling
- Dark urine

PROBLEMS FACED AFTER TREATMENT

— Overload of iron due to frequent blood transfusion
— Overload of iron can damage the endocrine system, liver, and heart
— If spleen has been removed, then the body is more susceptible to infections

PIECE OF ADVICE

— There is no harm in taking diets from a Dietitian, otherwise, you need to consult a doctor lifelong.
— Have a personalized diet.
— There is no treatment of major thalassemia but one can control the fluctuating levels of iron in the body.
— More of iron in the food
— Increase bone and muscle strength
— Moringa tea
— In major, have green tea after your meal

BOLD IS BEAUTIFUL
GIRL WITH THE WINGS

THALASSEMIA

Mridula, 19 years

"My body is not well; I feel so lethargic after some days. I need to go to the hospital for blood transfusion every 15 days. It's like I am living in a bad dream, in which I can't have fun for so many days at a stretch. After 10-11 days, I feel like I am not able to do anything. I feel tired, sleepy and my body starts aching and then, it is again time to go to the hospital. I can't dance for long and am not allowed to go on long trips with my friends," said Mridula, a teenage girl to me. I don't remember the last time I met such a bold and strong girl. She was 19 years old, college-going, who was independent, strong, and tough decision-maker. When I was talking to her, I was thinking how great her upbringing is. Her nature made a great place in my heart in our first meeting. When I asked any question to her mother, only Mridula replied because she knew everything and her parents had taught her to speak for herself.

"Since when are you facing this problem? Is anyone in your family thalassemic? How about the regularity of your menstrual cycle? What about your studies? Do you think it affects your mood or memory?" I asked a few questions to her.

"I am thalassemic since childhood, but that time the condition was not this severe and blood was transfused after every 1.5 or 2 months. But today, after every 15 days, my blood is transfused.

My grandmother was thalassemic, she was a minor one though. She didn't feel any kind of problem except that she was Anaemic after she delivered her children. About me, I don't get periods and yes, sometimes I feel that it affects my mood. I am a class topper so you can figure out my memory too (laughter). That's it about me and my family," she smiled.

"What is your dream, Mridula? What do you want to be?" I asked with curiosity, to know her mindset more.

She said very calmly, "I want to go to business school in London and want to pursue dance as my hobby / passion / happiness."

I have seen so many clients and patients in the last 13 years of my career but she was something different, she was blessed. Her aura was so positive, lively, and warm. She was an ambitious girl and a daydreamer. How come the universe is not allowing her to live her dreams?

I asked her to visit the clinic every 7th day, but she was a student at Chitkara University. She said that she will try to visit the clinic. I gave her the option of Sunday also if she was comfortable to come on Sunday. She had a sharp mind so I assumed that the treatment will be less problematic. Because every diet or medicine will work on the body only when the person is willing to get results and she was a highly positive person, so how come the law of attraction failed in her case.

I saw her reports of complete blood count (CBC), Haematocrit, Haemoglobin, Serum Iron, Ferritin, Transferrin, total iron-binding capacity (TIBC) etc. Her reports were bad and the levels were very low. Her condition was severe. I didn't hide anything from her because till that time, I had come to know her strength of handling the situations. She agreed to co-operate with me and we started our journey together.

I have planned more of nourishment in her diet, worked on her muscles, energy levels and asked her to start dancing. She was happy and took some positive hope from the clinic. She was with us for 8 months and recovered well. Blood transfusion was still there but after 2-3 months. She no longer felt lethargic after 10 days. Her blood test reports were getting better when we repeated her blood tests after three months. Haemoglobin did not increase at first but after sometime, it started rising. And after 8 months, her Haemoglobin was 11. She was the same strong girl who had wings on her back. She was preparing for her dream in London and simultaneously danced and flew.

When she came to us, her dietary chart was filled with burgers, pizza, or fried things as other teenagers but after 8 months, she was indeed habitual of healthy foodstuff. She knew the importance of beetroot, carrot, spinach, kiwi, pomegranate, ragi, jowar for her. I still remember her and teach Saadgi the same things which I learnt from that amazing girl. This girl didn't make me cry, be it with sadness or with happiness. But she made me strong enough to face any situation with a smile.

I wish everyone has sufficient gallons of blood flowing through their bodies with all the positive vibes.

Completely Yours, Dietitian Shreya!

OKAY, I AM CONVINCED

THALASSEMIA

Geetika, 32 years

I was excited because it was a small get-together at my house when I was 5 months pregnant with Shaurya. Our close relatives were coming from Jalandhar, Malerkotla, and Ambala. I am bad in figuring out the relation between people so everybody knew that I denoted young people as bhaiya bhabi and older people as uncle aunty, as it is easy to address them that way.

There was my bhabi (Geetika) who came to that party and we spoke about ladies' stuff like family, children, and work. She said, "My Haemoglobin is very low since childhood, cramps are severe during menstruation and conception was very tough too. But by God's grace, I got a baby boy. So what do you think, what should I have?" I heard her very carefully and suggested her many different things to take to increase her Haemoglobin. She said, "Okay, I will try them." I said, "I will help you out with this condition if you will help me by following the instructions." She was half-convinced and ignored the rest of it. Party finished; everyone went back to their native places but I wanted to stay in touch with my bhabi who lives in Malerkotla.

After 15 days, I got a call from her and she said, "Okay, I am convinced. Give me some suggestions about what should I do? I told her to have different things in this state and also asked her to lose some weight. Her weight was 80, low energy, pigmentation on the face, frequent headaches and she fainted sometimes. I planned her diet with light vegetables, fruits, salad, little of carbohydrate/fats and sweets.

After having diet for 2 months, there was less increase in the Haemoglobin. That was shocking to me. I asked her to do certain tests to confirm the problem and then, I got to know that she was thalassemic minor.

Her iron was very low; that was the reason for her symptoms. Her diet included pomegranate, kiwi, oranges, lemon, spinach, beetroot, mosami, ragi etc. More of vitamin C was given to her to increase the absorption in her body. I was concentrating more on her iron digits in the body rather than her weight or pigmentation on the face because everything is interconnected. When I started to work on her deficiencies of vitamins, it started to get better and iron-binding capacity increased. Her cramps during menstruation were less. Her bodyweight started reducing and her Hb improved by 12. I asked her to maintain this lifestyle for a lifetime or else the condition could get worse. She agreed and whenever she talks to me, I always say, 'Okay, I am convinced with your performance now' and laugh aloud.

Don't let Thalassemia hold you back, Fight against it and be the Superhero of your own life! So, I urge whosoever is reading this book to please donate blood and make your contribution towards life.

Sincerely Yours, Dietitian Shreya!

DIABETES..OUCH...

Prick It Before It Pricks You

INTRODUCTION

Diabetes is a condition in which the body fluctuates due to elevated blood sugar levels. There is an alteration in the carbohydrate, protein, and fat metabolism. As the body does not produce any or right amount of insulin, glucose remains in the blood and is not utilized properly by the body cells.

In some cases, the autoimmune system destroys the pancreatic cells leading to insulin deficiency (LADA - Latent Autoimmune Diabetes in Adults). Diabetes is considered a chronic condition. However, it can be managed and even reversed with the right lifestyle changes and diet.

There are three main types of Diabetes:

1) **Type 1 Diabetes/insulin-dependent Diabetes:** In this condition, the body is either producing less insulin or no insulin.

    Juvenile Diabetes is the name given to Type I Diabetes occurring in small children.

2) **Type 2 Diabetes:** It can be stress-induced or due to bad lifestyle choices. It can affect a person of any age but generally occurs in the middle-age of elderly people.

3) **Gestational Diabetes:** It develops in some women when they are pregnant. This kind of Diabetes generally goes away once the baby is born by following a good lifestyle. We can take care of it.

4) **LADA:** It can be related to a condition where the autoimmune system destroys the pancreatic cells leading to insulin deficiency. This is referred to as the latent autoimmune Disease of Diabetes.

The Disease is characterized by certain conditions known as hyperglycemia and hypoglycemia.

Hyperglycemia: Hyperglycemia or high blood sugar levels have serious long-term effects. This condition develops over several days or several weeks.

Hypoglycemia: It results due to the overdose of insulin/medication or not taking the meals on time. It may have serious consequences as low glucose can damage vital organs like brain, heart, and kidneys. It can lead to brain death, myocardial infarction, and can be fatal.

COMPLICATIONS ASSOCIATED WITH DIABETES

- **Diabetic nephropathy:** Prevalence of high blood sugar puts the pressure on the delicate filtering system of the kidneys. Patients of CKD may require dialysis and kidney transplant as the Disease progresses.

- **Neuropathy:** High blood sugar levels can lead to damage of blood vessels which nourish the nerves across the body, especially the legs. Patients feel a tingling sensation of burning pain. There is less sensation in the limbs and it also leads to digestion related issues like nausea, vomiting, and irregular bowel movements. If you are ignoring the symptoms, it can lead to Bell's palsy.

- **Glaucoma:** It is a condition whereby there is increased intraocular pressure leading to permanent vision loss. Apart from this, there can be damage to blood vessels in the retina and this can lead to a condition known as Diabetic Retinopathy.

- **Diabetic foot:** This is another problem arising out of nerve damage due to high blood sugar levels. Patients get cuts, blisters, and injuries that do not get cured. In the case of gas gangrene or infection in lower extremities, foot or leg amputation is required.

REASONS

- Autoimmunity
- Stress factor
- Family history of Diabetes
- During pregnancy
- Bad lifestyle
- Overweight

SYMPTOMS OF HYPOGLYCEMIA

- The affected person feels shaky and weak
- Pale skin
- Feel cold and clammy
- Confused, irritable, and irrational behaviour
- Palpitations & rapid pulse
- Loss of consciousness

SYMPTOMS OF HYPERGLYCEMIA

- Excessive thirst
- Frequent urination
- Abrupt weight loss
- Itchy skin
- Slow wound healing
- The patient may become drowsy leading to unconsciousness

DIAGNOSIS

Physical self-diagnosis

- Foam in urine
- Edema in lower extremities
- Discolouration of nails
- Slow wound healing
- Dark pigmentation on the feet
- Dark velvety skin around your neck, elbows, knuckles, and groin

TESTS

- Blood sugar level tests; fasting sugar, postprandial, and random
- HbA1c test (Haemoglobin glycosylated test): Average blood sugar of three months
- C-peptide (blood serum test): It determines if a person has Type I or type 2 Diabetes
- GAD 65 (glutamic acid decarboxylase test): This test helps in checking pancreatic cells, which gets destroyed in LADA.
- Renal function test
- Uric acid test
- GFR (glomerular filtration rate)
- Electrolytes (Na+, K+ and Cl-)

PIECE OF ADVICE

- Do check the blood sugar level in fasting, postprandial and random, especially, if you are carrying a family history of Diabetes

- Visit your Dietitian and doctor if you feel any of the above symptoms
- Avoid stress
- Avoid bakery products and refined sugar
- Take special care of weight management and keep a check on belly fat
- Stress-free life
- Small frequent meals
- Artificial laughter
- Set the biological clock by giving your stomach one food at a particular time
- Methi seeds powder half an hour before food helps in controlling the insulin resistance
- Jamun sirka before your second meal
- Barley has proven to be one miracle grain in controlling Diabetes
- Kachnar vegetable
- Avoid — potato, carrot, sweet potato, beetroot

WATERMELON SHAPED CUSHION

TYPE 1 DIABETES

Sara, 7 years

Mrs. Manju was a fashionista but this Monday, at 11:55 a.m., she visited in a dull olive-green suit. When I checked her form that week, she hadn't lost any weight even though she was a person committed towards her health. I could sense the sadness in her voice and even the fan's noise in the room was louder than her usual laughter.

Before I could ask her anything, she burst into tears and buried her reddened face into her palms. I rubbed my hand against her chilled fingers. "Shreya ma'am, I'm all broken today. My daughter, Sara, has been diagnosed with Type-I (Juvenile) Diabetes," said Mrs. Manju. No one could understand her pain like me as my daughter was also 7 then as Sara was. I remembered Sara as a little cute girl with curly hair and red was her favourite colour, as and when she used to enter my cabin, her first action was to directly jump on my red watermelon shaped cushions. "She is just 7 and a half, I can't let her take the unbearable pain of insulin injections," Mrs. Manju continued.

So, as I started telling Mrs. Manju that we can manage Sara's Diabetes with the right kind of food choice and that Sara didn't have any family history of Diabetes. As I am a strong believer in the law of attraction, my entire energy was working on Sara's wellness. I can't forget the next few words uttered by Mrs. Manju. "Ma'am, I am giving my own life in your hands now. I trust you and it feels like a stake in my chest, so please relieve us from this pain."

I was so determined in my mind that I had this aim to treat Sara's Type-I Diabetes. Her parents got all the medical tests done for Sara, including C-peptide. The good news was C-peptide was quite under range and we had possibilities to work on HbA1c which was 8.9. As Sara was a kid, the task was to make her understand the value of every meal she was putting in her mouth. So, I had to make sure that I plan healthy meals which had taste also. I started with a high protein diet and multi millet khichri and Amaranth porridge (Sara's favourites), she loved the almond milk. And we all were blessed with the way her body was responding. So, in the first quarter of the treatment, her fasting levels were improved from 225 to 120-140.

Now it was the time to get HbA1c done. So here it is Monday morning and I woke up with all the good wishes and blessings.

Around noon, I just gulped my salad juice as my mid-morning meal and realized that Sara hadn't visited the clinic yet, again I was engaged in my work and around 4 p.m., we received a message from Sara's mother that they won't be able to visit the clinic as Sara ate some sweets at her grandparents' house and her random sugar levels slightly went high so we had to delay the test for another week. But hard work always pays off and when I met Sara the next meeting, she brought a bouquet of red roses for me with the good news that her insulin had reduced to just 2 shots a day which was 4 shots previously.

I could see the tears of happiness in Mrs. Manju's eyes. This time, Mr. Anil, Sara's father was also present. Their smile was a true reward for me. After 4 more months, we achieved our target as Sara did not need to take any more insulin shots.

This particular case is so close to my heart that it makes my belief deeper in the law of attraction. This taught me a very important lesson that one decision can change your entire life, you can either make it or spoil it forever.

Take Away Tip: This girl has normal C-Peptide level and thus enough Insulin levels. That is the reason she managed to drop the artificial Insulin intake. There is no harm in taking controlled Diet than watching uncontrolled Sugars.

Affectionately Yours, Dietitian Shreya!

CLEAR WITH FLYING COLORS

TYPE I DIABETES

Ananya, 12 years

In the year 2014, I had started making videos on YouTube trying to reach and help more people. One of my diet workshops on women health videos went viral, as a result of which, lots of women started reaching out to me.

Simultaneously, my mother-in-law went for Satsang and one of the ladies there had shown her my videos on YouTube regarding healthy eating, Vitamin D deficiency, acidity, weight loss, and about kids. The videos were shared with other ladies in the Satsang Bhawan. Some of them asked my mother-in-law about Diseases like Diabetes, polycystic ovarian syndrome. My mother-in-law shared my contact number with them. After Satsang, one of the ladies made an appointment with me for her 12-year-old daughter, Ananya, who was suffering from Type I Diabetes Mellitus.

Ananya was studying in VIIIth standard and was a cheerful girl. Her health was the major concern of her parents. When I met her for the first time, she was so cheerful and mature at a tiny age.

Keeping that in mind, I had to draw a diet plan according to the physical and mental needs of a growing child. Another key factor to be considered was that she was on insulin injections as prescribed by a physician. I already had a success rate for diabetic people to maintain their blood sugar levels but this was my first case of juvenile Diabetes. I was challenged by this case and wanted to help Ananya like anything; to help her live like a normal child. Her HbA1c was 10 and her fasting sugar was 125 with insulin. I started her diet plan according to the timings of her school and asked her parents to talk to the teachers to let her eat in every 2 hours. I introduced eggs, channa, sattu, jaun, methi dana, jamun sirka, quinoa, kalonji in her diet plan and asked them to maintain a chart of blood sugar levels. Slowly, her blood sugar levels started getting lower to normal levels. She was happy with the way things were proceeding. Her HbA1c levels also landed at 6.5 from 10.

The family, as well as I, were grateful and we proceeded to talk to the concerned doctor regarding taking her off the insulin injections. Her doctor denied doing that bluntly on their face.

There seemed to develop a conflict between the doctor's idea of treatment and mine. I talked to the concerned doctor directly and asked him to at least consider my way of treatment. Even then the doctor strictly opposed my idea and I had to rely on the decision of her parents.

After talking to them and making them understand my perspective, Ananya's parents were ready to stop her insulin shots by reducing the dosage first and then completely took it off after six months of hard work. Her pancreas started to produce adequate insulin to keep the blood sugar levels at normal. This case is very near and dear to my heart as it serves as a testimony to the statement that no problem is too big to be solved.

Take Away Tip: You can reverse your Type 2 Diabetes under the guidance of your Clinical Dietitian but be cautious against gaining knowledge from Google or WhatsApp University.

Yours Diabetes Expert, Dietitian Shreya!

I AM HERE TO SURPRISE YOU

TYPE II DIABETES

Preeti, 44 years

It was a very special day for me as I was celebrating my clinic's 10th anniversary and I was so happy and could proudly say that I am at least able to make a small difference in the health sector. My videos were doing well on YouTube and people had started giving a great response to my social media accounts. Preeti was one of those people who visited the clinic after watching my video on "Diabetes Diet Plan by Dietitian Shreya." Preeti had a lot of darkness in life as she was a divorced mother with two daughters, Tanvi and Kriti. She had a lot of stress in her life and the cause was her being a single mother of two teens.

On our first meeting, Preeti told me about her grandmother who passed away due to Diabetic Nephropathy. So I got to know that she had a family history of Diabetes. "Even the thought of Diabetes makes me scared. I am already facing different challenges in my life. Life is giving me unbearable pain of loneliness, financial crisis, and the shadow of my shattered dreams," she said.

I asked her to show me her medical reports as she was already following a few tips from my videos and I noticed that, her initial HbA1c was 7.8. After a few weeks of observation, I concluded that her food choices were not to be blamed, because even when the carbohydrate intake was restricted, her fasting levels were not under control.

She used to stay up late at night, even her meal timings were not a priority for her. I suggested that Preeti should fix her meal timings and start doing deep breathing exercises at least twenty times a day and when I met Preeti in her next visit, I could see controlled diabetic chart levels.

Her fear for Diabetes was very obvious as she had seen her dearest grandmother who had to visit hospital almost every week for dialysis. Even after paying a hefty amount of money on medical bills for dialysis, they couldn't save her grandmother. She remembered the pain her grandmother went through during the procedure when the machine used to suck every drop of blood out of every single vein of hers.

As we achieved a controlled fasting chart, now we were aiming at our upcoming achievement, which was HbA1c, so I started planning more of Jaun sattu and egg in diets, which were rich in proteins as well as calcium for her bones. As a result, we achieved 5.4 HbA1c.

"I am here to surprise you!" Preeti exclaimed in our meeting when she showed me her reports and I was awarded one more successful result. She still visits after every quarter to show me her reports and her elder daughter also aspires to become a dietician. I just love it when even a single person gets their aspiration from me and my work.

"Kuch Aisa Kar Jao, Ki Tumahare Baad Bhi Duniya Tumhe Yaad Rakhe"

A MEET AND GREET

TYPE II & DIABETIC FOOT
Mrs. Harjinder Kaur, 54 years

Mrs. Harjinder Kaur had been suffering from Type II Diabetes for the last 15 years, her family had a very famous sweet shop in Moga.

On World Diabetes Day, I visited the Ludhiana clinic for "Meet and Greet". My first appointment of the day

was with her and she was visiting with her husband and her son.

I can still recall her elegant attire as she entered the counselling room. She had beautifully plaited long hair and was wearing a blue coloured Patiala suit and I noticed that Diabetes had started exhibiting its every possible physical symptom on her body. During the physical examination, I noticed that she had a deep black wound on her left foot which wasn't healing and her nails showed deep blue discolouration and they were so brittle. Her husband and her son were surprised as they had never noticed these symptoms and they always wondered about her rising blood glucose levels.

I questioned, "Ma'am, since how long do you have this wound?"

Mrs. Harjinder replied, "Eh tan aidan hi rehnda hai ." (This remains like this only.)

I was quite surprised that she had almost started forming diabetic foot and her attitude towards this was so ignorant. During such counselling sessions, I realized that there must be so many people around who are ignoring these symptoms like Mrs. Harjinder and I felt that I should work harder on making people aware about the same.

During the early days of internship at hospitals, many patients with diabetic foot used to visit. One such incident struck my mind after meeting Mrs. Harjinder Kaur. There was a lady who visited the hospital and was admitted on floor 2, bed number 56 and it was my turn to visit all the beds and check patient meals. She had a striking resemblance with my massi, so I went up to her and had a small conversation with her. She complimented me for my hair and her voice was so soothing and calming. After examining her meals, I called it a day and the very next day was a holiday. And when I joined back, I saw that her leg had been amputated because of excessive damage caused by Diabetes. That day I realized that I can save many people just by making changes in their lifestyle before it's too late.

When I asked Mrs. Harjinder Kaur for her average glycated test (HbA1c), she told me, "Haemoglobin tan theek hi rehnda hai mera." (My Haemoglobin level remains normal). I replied, "Ma'am, yeh aapka teen mahine ka blood glucose levels ka average hota hai jis se aapke Diabetes status ka pata chalta hai" (HbA1c is an average blood glucose level of three months which gives an idea about how well your Diabetes is being controlled). Her family was also not aware of these tests. Her son showed me the test reports that were done at the doctor's suggestion; her HbA1c was 8.2. It was high time to work on this otherwise any moment the doctor could put her on insulin shots.

During the meeting she told me about her daily dietary recall, her morning started with a cup of tea and biscuits and she used to consume wheat chapatti, rice with all the possible starchy vegetables (aloo, arbi ki sabzi etc.). She also gained approximately 15 kilograms of extra weight.

Now my focus was very clear. We needed to work on the inches around her abdomen. As winters were approaching, I planned channa sattu and pearl millet in her diet. I was giving her methi dana every day, in the grounded form with hot water and added plenty of proteins in her diet. She had low vitamin D3 levels, so we made sure that she sits in sunlight for at least 15 minutes a day before 11 a.m.

After 4 months, I received a medicine drop box picture from the clinic and Mrs. Harjinder was looking completely transformed; she had lost 12 kilograms and her medicine had been dropped with her doctor's prescription as her HbA1c was 5.6 now. Her family gave me a surprise visit at my Chandigarh clinic with my favourite kaju katli box.

This story is inspiring to me as I saw the same lady in Harjinder Kaur, whom I met at the hospital and I thanked God that he chose me as a saviour.

Yours Saviour, Dietitian Shreya!

MILK, TWO CUPS A DAY

GESTATIONAL DIABETES

Anupama, 25 years

Every day I learn something new and my motive behind my karma is helping people and giving them the gift of knowledge. One such lesson came to me from Anupama. She belongs to a small town based at Himachal and I was already amazed at the distance she had covered to meet me. This was such a pure and loving gesture. At that time, I had also shed off my post-partum weight after the birth of Shaurya, my son, and was running a challenge for all the new mothers. Anupama checked the challenge on Facebook and messaged me on messenger; hence, we met each other.

Anupama and Rajiv tied the knot two years back and now the most beautiful phase of their life had started. Anupama had conceived and it was the beginning of her second trimester. Pregnancy is a beautiful transformation for a female but Anupama was quite stressed as she was diagnosed with Gestational Diabetes.

When I was reading her form, I carefully checked, Anupama was eating two pinnis daily and as per the rituals at her place, she had to drink Ghee or Milk, two cups a day. She told me that her mother-in-law makes sure whether she was having all the nutrition or not. It brought many thoughts to my mind as she was lacking complete nutrition in her diet.

She was asked by a doctor to take 2 insulin shots daily because of Gestational Diabetes and I recommended her to stick to 1200Kcal intake. As per her family, she was taking complete nutrition but as per my calculations, she wasn't even consuming half of the nutrition required. Her body needed many micronutrients with her major meals.

I introduced ragi in her diet which has more calcium than milk and for good iron intake, I planned palak soup in her meals, also included makhana in her diet. I spoke to her mother-in-law over the call so that there will be no eating restrictions for Anupama. Initially, her family wasn't as convinced as Anupama was. But as I always believe, results speak better. Her fasting levels were quite under control after maintaining her lifestyle and finally, her family was happy.

Today, she is a beautiful mother of an angelic daughter and now she is taking post-partum diet and hasalready lost 7 kilograms in 2 months.

And her journey continues with us through our guidance and tips on our YouTube channel and other social media handles.

Forever Digitally Yours, Dietitian Shreya!

WILL BE HOME ON TIME

GESTATIONAL DIABETES

Kritika, 29 years

Kritika is the daughter of a famous businessman from Chandigarh, Mr. Deepak Ahluwalia. She is now married to Mr. Abhinav Mahajan. Mr. Deepak visits my clinic from the starting days of my clinic and thus, his entire family has visited us for their diet.

Kritika had been a bubbly girl who used to visit with her father and used to tell me about every little cheat meal her father was consuming during his weight loss journey. But this time when they entered the counselling room, Mr. Deepak seemed to be little nervous and Kritika wasn't as bubbly as she used to be. It was for the first time I was meeting her after her marriage a duration of almost 1.5 years. She was pregnant and had grown up into a beautiful lady. She started narrating her last visit to her gynaecologist. "I am 20 weeks pregnant now and have been diagnosed with Gestational Diabetes, even Papa is diagnosed with a pre-diabetic condition so I am a little worried for our child."

She held my hand in hers and said, "Shreya ma'am, you are my biggest hope. Because you treated my father, I know you can also treat me. I am in love with every little moment of pregnancy, it has completely changed me, from immaturity to the sense of responsibility, and it is teaching me everything. Just this one thing is pulling me back. I am fed up of pricking my finger again and again. During pregnancy, I am already having these mood blues and sometimes I hate checking on my blood sugar levels…"

I explained to Kritika that usually most of the females get rid of Gestational Diabetes after delivery; she just needs to be more particular about her meals and lifestyle. "Ma'am, I wait for Abhinav as he reaches home around 11 p.m. I have a habit of taking my meals with him, so how do I manage my meals?" she said.

Before I could say anything, Abhinav said, "I'll make this change; as our child is not only your responsibility. I will be home on time from now on."

She is blessed to have a supportive family as many females lack such support from their respective families and end up harming themselves or their child.

I asked her to consume 4 to 5 portions of salads and fruits every day. As she could consume eggs, I recommended her to consume at least 4-5 egg whites daily, 10-20 grams of fats was given to her on daily basis (in her diet), and we avoided refined sugar and shifted to Stevia. I increased her intake of folic acid, calcium and iron in the food groups. Chia seeds were an important part of her dietary regime as they are rich in all micronutrients and proteins.

This diet brought her blood glucose levels under control and now the family is blessed with a baby boy, Ryan Mahajan. I have celebrated every moment with Mr. Deepak so I was invited at Ryan's Annaprasan and I was honoured to make him eat his first meal — coconut water in a silver container. This is the only treasure of mine, which I am earning every day.

Take Away Tip: EAT RIGHT DIET, BITE BY BITE

Sweet Always, Yours, Dietitian Shreya!

THYROID

Let The Butterfly "Fly"

INTRODUCTION

The impaired function of the butterfly-shaped gland that sits low on the front of the neck can cause a Disease called Thyroid. The Thyroid has two side lobes, connected by a bridge (isthmus) in the middle. When the Thyroid is in its normal size, you can't feel it. It can be due to iodine deficiency or can be an autoimmune Disorder either hyper or Hypo Thyroid.

Hypo Thyroid — It happens when the gland does not make enough Thyroid hormones (T3 and T4). It is also an underactive and a non-functioning Thyroid.

CAUSES OF HYPO THYROID

- Hyper Thyroid treatment (radioiodine)
- Radiation treatment of certain Cancers
- Thyroid removal
- Auto Immune Disorder

SYMPTOMS OF HYPO THYROID

- Feeling cold more than other people
- Constipation
- Weakness and pain in muscles
- Weight gain
- Feeling sad, depressed, and tired
- Pale, dry skin
- Thinning of hair
- Slow heart rate

- A hoarse voice
- More bleeding in periods

DIAGNOSIS

- Blood tests (Thyroid test)
- Physical symptoms

HYPER THYROID

Hyper Thyroid or overactive Thyroid causes your Thyroid to make more Thyroid hormone than your body needs. This speeds up many of your body's functions like your metabolism and heart rate.

SIGNS AND SYMPTOMS

- Weight loss, even if you eat the same or more food (most but not all people lose weight)
- Eating more than usual
- Rapid or irregular heartbeat or pounding of your heart
- Feeling nervous or anxious
- Feeling irritable
- Trouble sleeping
- Trembling in your hands and fingers
- Increased sweating
- Feeling hot when other people do not
- Muscle weakness
- Diarrhea or more bowel movements than normal
- Fewer and lighter menstrual periods than normal
- Changes in your eyes that can include bulging of the eyes, redness, or irritation

CAUSES

Autoimmune Disorder (Graves' Disease)

DIAGNOSIS

— Physical examination
— Medical history
— Blood tests
— Thyroid scan or ultrasound

HASHIMOTO'S DISEASE

The most common cause of Hypo Thyroid is Hashimoto's Disease. In people with Hashimoto's Disease, the immune system mistakenly attacks the Thyroid gland. This attack damages the Thyroid so that it does not make enough hormones. It occurs due to the age factor, family history of Thyroid or autoimmune Disorder. Hashimoto's Disease induces destruction of the Thyroid gland. It is diagnosed with the presence of goiter with high TSH levels and by the test of Anti-TPO.

GRAVES' DISEASES

Graves' Disease is the most common cause of Hyper Thyroid. For reasons that remain unknown, it is more common in women, particularly those aged 30–50. It affects approximately 3% of women and 0.3% of men. Graves' Disease is associated with abnormalities of the eyes and integument.

Bulging eyes and puffy eyelids and, certainly, eye Disease is frequently associated with it. It can be due to environ mental factors or genetically transferred from ancestors. In this, one can face tiredness, weight gain, weakness in muscles, and pain in joints, depression, mood swings and mental confusion. It can be diagnosed by blood tests, physical examination, imaging tests etc.

PIECE OF ADVICE

- Stress-free life
- Artificial laughter
- Have your last meal before sunset
- Gluten-free diet
- High protein
- Red onion juice with lukewarm water in mid-morning. Honey can be added to help stimulate the gland to produce Thyroid hormone
- Brazil nuts are effective in the stimulation of hormone.

FLORAL PASTEL COLOR DRESS

THYROID

Aastha, 28 years

Aastha had just finished with a project at her company and was about to start a new phase of life. It was her engagement and she started feeling huge changes in herself. She started feeling anxiety, tiredness, and fatigue. She thought it to be because in the new start of life or maybe she was just nervous. But eventually, all these symptoms were increasing and now she had started having hair fall and mood swings also.

So she decided to get her blood tests done, where she found out that her TSH levels were around 9. Her doctor suggested her to start with medicine after anti-TPO test or diet. She chose diet over medicine and searched online for Dietitian and got my clinic's contact details.

As she was also suggested to get her anti-TPO tests done, her doctor didn't start with the medicines till then.

As she told me, she was not having any family history of Hypo Thyroid so we had good chances to treat it.

We started working on her body with gluten-free diets and I asked her to do deep breathing exercises, as Thyroid patients tend to get frequent mood swings and hair fall also. I needed to plan foods rich in Sulphur, so I started planning diluted red onion juice in her diet and boiled green coriander with jeera water.

We had another 3 months for her engagement and we started on a positive note. It was a stubborn wish and it had to be successful. During our further conversations, I got to know that she was under stress and was trying to maintain a balance in her personal and professional life as she wanted to move abroad for professional goals and her family wanted her to get married. So, I asked her to go slow with her emotions as her sleepless and disturbed nights could be the reason for elevated TSH levels.

Chamomile tea proved to be a great support for her and within those next three months, it was a miracle that her TSH levels came down to 4.8.

She wore such a beautiful floral pastel-coloured dress on her engagement and got married soon with a healthy body and a calm mind. Now she has moved to Sydney as her husband got a project there, and now she can be more focused on her career goals.

Not less, not more, let it be balanced!

Dietitian Shreya!

PRACTICE WHAT YOU PREACH

THYROID

Mrs. Amarjyoti Tripathi, 45 years

Mrs. Amarjyoti Tripathi visited my clinic when her weight was 84 kgs and she was diagnosed with the early stages of Hypo Thyroid. She got to know about my clinic through a colleague. I remember she was a school principal but her confidence was very low.

She was suffering from severe pains in her entire body. After some time, it became almost impossible for her to move from bed; moreover, her personal life was tough. While I was asking her for the symptoms, she told me usually she didn't feel any severe kind of fatigue, hair fall or stress.

Suddenly, she started gaining weight and was entering into an anxious lifestyle. Then she decided to get her medical reports done, she was diagnosed to have Hypo Thyroid and before rushing to an endocrinologist, she wanted to give a try to better her lifestyle and diet. We got her Anti-TPO diagnosed and as per that she was on the safer side as it was not an auto-immune Disorder.

Practice what you preach. She was a perfect example of discipline to her students. She had elevated cholesterol levels with Hypo Thyroid; hence, it was supposed to be a diet low in fats, high in proteins and fiber, and completely gluten-free.

She had been associated with me from the past 3 years and in between, she was diagnosed with PCOD, as this hormonal imbalance was inherited from her grandparents. So, we decided to go gluten-free again and started with all the possible precautions.

She touched 69 kgs and is now doing skin diet and leading a beautiful life without Hypo Thyroid, PCOD, and high cholesterol. With her results, she inspired many; she even gave a video for my YouTube channel.

Age is just a number, Enjoy every moment!

Always at your service, Dietitian Shreya!

GLINT IN THE EYES

HASHIMOTO DISEASE

Mohsin, 40 years

2017, I was on a trip to Dubai and already had one or two meetings lined up with my dear clients, so I decided to keep a short meet and greet session there. Mohsin was among some visiting people. When Mohsin entered the hotel room, her beautiful eyes stood out of all the features as she was wearing a black beaded burkha. She was soft-spoken, as she wished, "Good afternoon."

During that meeting, we had every possible discussion on people back there in India, shopping in Dubai, and local dishes. While having this conversation, I noticed that Mohsin had to clear her throat several times. When I checked her reports her TSH was shooting to 36 ug/dL and her doctor got her anti-TPO done; sadly, it was also raging high.

She spoke about her experience with Hashimoto's as doctors had already suggested her to remove the gland. "I have a beautiful family, a supportive husband, and a lovely kid and still my anxiety has no boundaries.

Many a times I start shouting, yelling at my family and then I realize that I'm doing something wrong. In the mornings, it becomes a task to move out of the bed; it feels like I am carrying hundred kilos of weight from ages and now I am tired. Ma'am, I am at a point where I get thoughts of mercy-killing." Her words gave me chills throughout my spine.

I gave her a warm hug and offered a cup of lemon water. I felt like pulling out all the pain and suffering from her life, but we needed to have patience as it was not a matter of one or two days. Coming over to her lifestyle, I got to know that she was continuously having bakery and cruciferous food. Even without any consultation, she was using black salt in her diet that meant she was avoiding iodine in her diet unintentionally.

So, my first question was, "Do you want to get rid of these pains?" And suddenly, I saw a glint in her eyes; she said, "That's my dream." I continued, "Dear, it's all in your head and if you are going to have any negative thoughts in your mind regarding your health, no source can ever give a solution for this. So have faith in nature; it will take away your pains."

So, we started our journey there, majorly, I planned gluten-free food for her that had Licorice and Ginseng along. I recommended her to take continuous steam and sauna, along with bathing salt baths. She was completely off bakery and bread, for her it is a lifestyle which can keep all the pains away and now she is running a boutique there, setting an example for many.

Versatility shines only when you shine! Keep yourself healthy, keep shining

Dietitian Shreya!

RAVAIYA; THE BEHAVIOUR

GRAVES' DISEASE

Kirti, 17 years

Kirti visited my Chandigarh clinic, accompanied by her mother. She was wearing blue pants with a black half-sleeved T-shirt. Her physical appearance indicated that she was not well by health — her eyes were bulging out and was having a goiter around her throat. She was weighing 38 kgs then and her height was 152 cm.

As I read her prescription card from the hospital, I got to know that she had Graves' Disease. So I started with general questioning about her health as her mother interrupted our conversation and said,"Madamji, yeh kuch khaati peeti hi nahi hai, hum toh pareshan ho gye hain iske is raviye se." (Ma'am, she doesn't eat anything; we are tired of her behavior.)

Kirti's card was saying that she also had depression and was consuming anti-depressants for the same. She was also concerned for her entrance exam and wasn't even getting enough sleep. I wanted to make her aware of the situation, as she had been avoiding this for a long time, so she started with a trial diet. Unfortunately, her family didn't have much faith in the right kind of lifestyle and Disease management. So, the first hurdle for her good health was her family's thinking.

We started the diet, we had to cut down on lactose and gluten, but due to ignorance, her family kept on giving her milk and ghee every day, despite knowing that Graves' has started affecting her heart. Apart from this, she was diagnosed with early age Osteoporosis and I saw her hands trembling badly. But even after hours of counselling, her family wanted to feed her with all the calories loaded fats.

When I tried to oppose their decision, they took Kirti from the middle of the counselling and told me that she was not getting better by medicines so how could I help her. So, it was better not to waste time and left the cabin abruptly. That day I felt very bad for Kirti because I knew that this would badly affect her health.

A few weeks had passed but that incident was still in my mind, right in front of my eyes. It was Saturday and a busy day at the clinic, but my team managed to call Kirti's mother just to ask about her health but in return, I received a message that Kirti is hospitalized in emergency. "It was her heart that failed her". I couldn't help her and she had to pay for it by losing her own precious life. I was stunned and felt empty from inside. I wish her family could have been more supportive of her health and lifestyle.

It was a sad day for me and my team but I still wanted to share this with you so that such conditions would not be ignored.

Take Away Tip: 10% is what happens to you and 90% is how you react to it.

With all Positive vibes, Dietitian Shreya!

TYPHOID

Not So Cool

Typhoid fever is caused by Salmonella Typhus. Infection is caused by the intake of food contaminated with the pathogen, transmission through unhygienic conditions and sewage contamination. Some symptoms are body aches, headache, sweating, dry cough, fever, weakness, abdominal pain, and diarrhea. Symptoms vary from mild to severe and life-threatening. It can be detected by a test called Vidal test which can be done with a blood sample.

PIECE OF ADVICE

- Wash your hands to prevent infection
- Avoid drinking untreated water
- Avoid having raw food and packaged food
- Choose hot and properly cooked food
- Have steaming chicken soup, sheera, and more of liquids
- Work on Immunity.
- It's just a phase of life and it will pass, don't worry.

A GOOD COMPANY

TYPHOID

Aasha, 26 years

Aasha is a sweet, caring, and lovable girl in my office. Her nature to talk to everyone amiably is captivating. If anyone is angry, she can make him/her smile with her happy soul. She stays calm and works for the betterment of people. When I took her interview,

I found her quite untangled and emotional too. This attracted me towards her and now she is in my office for 2 years. She has been also very connected to my son, Shaurya. When he comes to the clinic, Aasha plays with him and makes him laugh. I must say, she has earned many blessings from people in and outside the clinic. But sometimes, blessings work after a certain time.

One day I was in the clinic and heard sounds of coughing again and again. I went to my team and asked who was not well. They told me that Aasha was not feeling well from the past two days. I asked her what happened. She said, "I am allergic to dust, so maybe this is due to the dust." That was Diwali time and everywhere, the cleaning process was going on. So, I asked her to shift to some other cabin which had gone through the cleanliness process already.

The next day her cough was bad, like very bad, with severe body ache. I asked her to go back and take some rest. But she refused and said, "I will be alone in my apartment, my roommate is not in town so what will I do there? I am okay and you all are here. If I faint, at least you all will take care of me." I prepared turmeric ginger tea and besan halwa for her so that her body aches and throat would feel better. She had it and took rest for a while in the cabin. Her throat was good after having that but her body temperature elevated. She was shivering badly since morning. I asked Ravi, our data analyst, to take her to the doctor. The doctor suggested some blood tests like jaundice, typhoid, dengue, malaria, etc. When her blood test reports showed up, we were shocked. Her typhoid titer value was quite high, 80:160 and she was Anaemic too, which made her weak. I was not able to see her in that much pain and asked her to shift with me for a few days. I asked her to do so because she was alone in the apartment and her parents were in Canada, so no one was there to take care of her. At first, she refused but somehow, I convinced her.

Her body was weak, so I planned her diet accordingly. I gave instructions to Vikas, my cook, to prepare easy to digest food (more of rice, soup, millets, eggs), more fruits (especially pomegranate and kiwi) and turmeric ginger teas to fight with the bacteria Salmonella typhus. I added Immunity boosting supplements and tea-like spirulina and moringa to her daily routine. She caught these bacteria from the water in her apartment as the water purifier had not been repaired. So, I took care of each and everything for her to make her feel comfortable and healthy.

She was recovering fast and was happy to be there too. We used to sit together every night and talk about books and music. Sometimes, only some good company and conversation can help in recovery. We repeated her tests and found her titer was normal. I was happy that she was healthy now but at the same time, I was sad and felt emotional that she was going back to her apartment; it was like Saadgi is moving out from home. But it was destined. I gave her my blessings and healthy food so that she would not face the pain again, that she had faced. We meet in the clinic daily and find the same late-night chit-chat bond in between.

It's not just the bacteria that spreads the infection, sometimes it's the polluted mind too! Stay Positive, Stay Hygienic!

Positively Yours, Dietitian Shreya!

FIRST ROAD TRIP

TYPHOID

Riya, 31 years

I constantly believe that we need to reach out to needy people so that they can acquire help on time. People are losing optimism, tranquility, and wealth on those things which they are unaware of. For example, if they choose more antibacterial, antiviral or Immunity booster food items throughout the seasonal change, then they can be saved from many Diseases. To make people attentive, we give different digital diet tips like acidity, Bp, viral, insomnia, etc. With these diet tips, we always provide our contact number, email address, and postal address, which helps people to approach us easily.

Due to these diet tips, there were two visitors in the clinic, they did not want any diet plan; they just entered to get answers to their questions. They came early in the clinic, so my team member, Shaheen, met them.

When Shaheen entered the cabin to meet them, they were already sitting there and they were looking a bit stressed. Shaheen introduced herself and asked about them. "I am Inderpreet Kaur, he is my husband, Vishal and we are here for our daughter, Riya and she is the only child we have." They were asking some strange questions like confused, helpless, and hopeless parents. "Please tell us first, how can you cure typhoid with diet? She gets inflected with typhoid after every 4/5 months and she has been suffering with this issue for the past 3 years. Hume bas yahi janna hai ki aap log kya karte ho? Kya khane ko dete ho? Jo hum nahi de rahe hai use." Shaheen calmed them down and made them understand the importance of right diet, healthy lifestyle, and education. Shaheen asked them many questions about her age, birth, medical conditions, personal life, and hygienic conditions but they did not answer properly. They wanted our help but simultaneously stopped us from helping them.

I came to the clinic to start my day. Shaheen was inside with the clients and she instructed Aarti, our office coordinator, to inform her when I get to the clinic. Shaheen asked them to wait for a while and came to meet me. She explained everything about Riya and her parents. Based on her description, I demanded to meet them personally.

They met me with a stressed mind, small fake smile, and warm greetings. I did not ask anything about their daughter at first and just asked about them. To know a little more about Riya's concern, I asked them a few questions. "Did you both have any medical condition in the past or present? Did you face any problem during pregnancy?" However, I did not ask directly; otherwise, I would have not got the answer. At first, they were hesitating. I asked again and again (I was looking like a cunning person to them but that was the only way I had). Lastly, they broke the silence with tears in their eyes. I said sorry to God for being so unsympathetic sometimes. They held each other's hand, looked into each other's eyes and started telling me about the past. I offered them a glass of water and was listening to them very carefully.

They had faced a lot of struggle in life: they were from different religions but they fell in love, they got married against the norms of society and families. She was a Sikh and he was from a Hindu family; the main concern of her family was the land owned by him as in Sikh culture, parents look for land as security to marry their girls. They ran from the house to get married and later were abandoned by their families which they had already predicted, so, to make a living, they moved to a different city.

"When I got pregnant, we thought they will accept us but they did not. And that made us feel very bad. I was much tensed during my pregnancy. We were not that rich to fulfil nutrition as well, but we have given our best to our child. She got delivered as a premature baby and the doctor put her under observation for 48 hours. In the early stage, the baby got infected with jaundice and I got an infection in my stitches, but the biggest challenge was that my mammary glands were not secreting milk to feed her. We tried everything, asked doctors, went to gurudwaras and temples but nothing helped us.

Time passed on and we promised that we will protect her from every problem in life. From her childhood, she was very susceptible to cough, cold, viral or any kind of infection. Doctors told us that her Immunity was very low because she did not cross the microflora of your vagina due to C- section and did not get colostrum (mother's milk), and there were other reasons too for her not having good Immunity. We decided to guard her against every infection by taking care of her. She grew up as a good-looking young girl and fell for a Sikh guy from Bathinda. We were not too impressed with the guy but we still remember the struggles that we had in our own time and accepted her happiness. After their marriage, she got frequent viral infections, cough, cold, jaundice, typhoid, body aches, etc. We told him to take good care of her and to take proper precautions but they ignored and it only got worse with time. It turned into a nightmare for her when at the age of 31, he left her by stating, she is not in good shape and all his hard-earned money is being wasted on her medicines.

She is having typhoid from the past three years which is reoccurring after every 4 months. Doctors have tried the best but it keeps reoccurring.

Her story gave me goosebumps and with all my courage, I asked them, "Where is she? Can I meet her?" They replied she is in Ropar at home. Immediately, I asked, "Can I go and meet her?" They were shocked and said, "Yes, of course!" I instantly asked my driver and Feroza from my team to join me in visiting her the very next day.

We got there to meet her. She was a young beautiful lady and even after facing so much in life, she looked so calm, positive, and chulbuli. I felt very bad when I saw her lying in bed due to weakness. She asked me, "So are you my new doctor? Hi, I am Riya!" I said, "No, I am not your doctor. I am your friend, Riya, and we will have fun together." I smiled and winked. While shaking hands with her, I found her very weak, with dark circles under her eyes. I asked some important questions like 'Where were you at the time when you got typhoid infection?' 'What were you eating?' She was not able to recall everything because 3 years is a long time but she told me a few things. Feroza and I discussed some points and started her diet plan.

We planned more of liquids, more of Immunity-boosting food, especially for typhoid. When she got her titer controlled, I started her diet for Immunity, strength, muscles, bones, IQ, and skin, like more of protein, micro, and macronutrients. She was with me for a year but during her journey, she got some infections, however, the severity of those was very less. More than this, I am glad for her parents and her dreams. She wanted to be a hippie-like person who could roam around everywhere happily and she went on her first road trip to Manali with her parents and gifted me with a very beautiful picture which she had clicked. And that picture is in my diary and always reminds me that life is beautiful.

Life is really beautiful, value it, by valuing your health!

Lovingly Yours, Dietitian Shreya!

CHRONIC OBSTRUCTIVE PULMONARY DISEASE (COPD)

Don't Let The Obstruction Block The Way

COPD is a progressive lung Disease that hinders airflow and makes it uneasy to Breath. COPD is (currently) an incurable Disease; however, can be prevented. With the right diagnosis and management, one can manage their COPD and breathe better. COPD can cause coughing, mucus production, wheezing, shortness of breath, chest tightness, and other symptoms. Exposure to lung irritants for a longer period, smoking, air pollution or dust and fumes can be responsible for COPD.

PIECE OF ADVICE

— Increased shortness of breath
— Frequent coughing (with or without mucus)
— Increased breathlessness
— Wheezing
— Tightness in the chest
— Punish the culprit, not your lungs
— Spirometry exercises
— Avoid polluted air by planting more trees

THE BREATH

COPD

Jaysee, 21 years

Before Christmas, Feroza messaged me that a girl named Jaysee wants to meet me urgently and she is coming from Ludhiana. I told her that she can visit the Ludhiana clinic as there is no need to visit here and if there will be some serious issue, diet counsellors will call me for that. Feroza forwarded my message to Jaysee but she refused to visit Ludhiana and said that she wishes to meet me in particular, as she is going back to her home town, Dehradun.

I said okay and the appointment was fixed for December 24, 2017. She was the only appointment on that day in the early hours of the clinic.

"I am a student of DMC Ludhiana, doing MBBS from there. I am going back to Dehradun for Christmas and New Year, so my sister Sharon suggested me to visit you in between regarding the problem I am having. Your people had visited Dehradun, so my sister met them for my issues. She was quite convinced by your work, therefore, I am here" she told me, "Being in a medical stream, I know the importance of healthy food in life and I also know that my problem will not be 100% cured but I want to control it badly," she continued.

When she was talking, she wheezed a lot in between, her voice was heavy and breath was short. She was suffering from a chronic obstructive pulmonary Disease (COPD); her cough was thick and and felt pain and tightness in the chest. Her condition was not this severe before entering Ludhiana.

Ludhiana is polluted and in winters, smog increases in the surrounding which causes difficulty in breathing and increases cough.

"When I cry a lot, I need to take injections to control my condition. Can you help me with this condition? Is it controllable?" Jaysee asked curiously.

I told her, "Yes, it is possible to control your severe situation. Yes, it will not be 100% cured but we can control it in certain ways like you should use a mask when you go out for anything. Try to avoid any kind of smell like deodorant or perfumes, try to plant more trees around your house, avoid places where smoking is normal. Have lukewarm water, broccoli, eggs, turmeric ginger tea; also try to avoid curd, lemon, and apple cider vinegar in your daily routine." I told her not to visit the Chandigarh clinic and visit the Ludhiana clinic after coming back from her native place.

When I came back from my vacation of Christmas and New year, I met her again and was glad to know that the persistence of attack was a bit slow, not slower or completely controlled but we were on the right path and we had achieved our destination at the end of May when she got used to the precautions and diet.

After knowing this kind of condition, I always feel that we need to plant more and more trees around our houses, parks, and roads. It will help us breathe and will give life to nature.

Take Away Tip: Value Your Lungs

Yours, Dietitian Shreya!

OUR DELHI

COPD

Sweta, 60 years

As we celebrate every important day for mankind; we were also celebrating national pollution prevention day on December 2, 2018. And in India, if we talk about pollution, then we cannot neglect Delhi. For that exposure, we were travelling via metro from Rohini to Rajiv Chowk in October. We were noticing each and everything around us. People were wearing masks on their faces due to the smog. When we looked outside the window, it was all blurred. The level of pollution was increasing day-by-day and not only in Delhi but also in Ludhiana, Bangalore, Varanasi, Patna and the list continues. When I visited the clinic in Delhi,

I met many people over there. I met 10 people in the clinic and 4 of them were facing asthma and COPD. Not only smog or pollution but smoking cigarettes is also a major trigger of this Disease. Kids, adults, and aged people, no one is untouched from COPD or asthma.

I met Sweta regarding the same, she was taking diet from our clinic for the last 3 weeks. When I met her, I asked her concern as COPD was mentioned in the form. Her age was 60 years and she was dealing with this problem for the last 15 years majorly. She was facing severe nasal blockage, excessive sneezing in the morning, shortness of breath and felt tightness in the chest after a run or a jog. She was all fit and was very enthusiastic about all the physical activities but one thing which was pulling her back was her COPD. Her diet started for COPD but some tiny points were missing in that.

I mentioned doing some spirometry exercises, using masks as people usually use in the metro, planting more trees (which is important for everyone), having less citrus, more heat-producing food, avoiding curd and having more of protein in the diet.

After a few weeks, I took Sweta's contact number from the clinic and called her up to inquire about her progress. She told me, these small things which I mentioned to her were very helpful. She can now go for a walk with her grandchildren and enjoy small moments in her life. She used to keep her inhaler with her but after taking the precautions and diet, now she uses it less. She invited me to join the Tree Delhi organization with her so that we could make aware people regarding pollution, trees, and these kinds of precautions. I was happy that people are taking this kind of initiative for the prevention of pollution and leading a healthy life.

Take Away Tip : Value Nature, Own a Plant!

Healthily Yours, Dietitian Shreya!

JAUNDICE

Yellow Yellow, Dirty Fellow

When red blood cells break down in the body, it forms bilirubin. If its concentration increases, it leads to jaundice and shows the symptom like yellow tint in the eyes and skin or dark urine. Also, an inflamed liver can lead to jaundice.

The diagnosis of jaundice can involve a range of tests. Numerous healthy babies have some jaundice in the first week of their life. It typically goes away. However, jaundice can happen at any age.

Jaundice occurs due to many reasons, such as:

— Blood Diseases
— Genetic syndromes
— Liver Diseases, such as hepatitis or cirrhosis
— Blockage of bile ducts
— Infections
— Medicines

PIECE OF ADVICE

— Jaundice does not cure by a broom; for that, you need to take care of liver and bilirubin levels
— High carbohydrate diet
— High-fat diet
— Avoid proteins in the diet

WORLD TOUR

JAUNDICE

Adamaya, 23 years

"Hello! I am Aparna from Yamunanagar. Can I get an appointment for tomorrow i.e. May 25, 2018, at 3:30 p.m. to meet Dietitian Shreya? Please, it's a bit urgent for me to meet her," a lady called my team and said. My team replied, "Shreya Ma'am's appointment slot is already booked for tomorrow but we can fix the appointment for May 26." The lady denied to wait and said, "It's okay. I will wait for her or I can wait in the waiting area for as long as it takes for her to make time for me." When my team told me about this lady, I agreed to meet her.

She came on the exact date on time but as she knew that it will take time, she was prepared for that. As it was Friday and we were also preparing to celebrate the World Environment Day on June 5, some meetings were also going on. She had waited for 30-40 minutes and then the time to meet her came. I rang the bell from the cabin and asked Aarti to send her in. A young lady entered the cabin, her hair was red-black and shining and her body was perfectly toned, but her face was pale and her movement was slow. She said hi with a small smile as she was tired of talking already. She was looking weak to me. I asked, "So, you are Aparna, right?" No, I am Adamaya. Aparna is my mother, she got a phone call from home and will join us in a while, "she said calmly.

"Okay then! Can we start or should we wait for your Mumma?" I asked humbly. She said, "The concern is mine, so yeah! We can start, she will come." I just asked her to introduce herself. "As you know my name, I am Adamaya, 23-years-old working in TCS, Delhi."

"Sorry for interrupting but why do you look so pale, your eyes are also pale and tired? What is your concern, Adamaya?" I asked. Her mother entered and said, "Sorry, got an urgent phone call. Hi, I am Aparna, her mother. I called you yesterday for an appointment for my daughter. Actually, Adamaya ki kuch dino ki chutti thi to ghar aagyi, iska face hume bohut pila lag raha tha to humne iske blood test karvaliye, you also have a look. "She told me everything in one go and she looked very tensed.

"How is your drinking habit, Adamaya?" I asked her directly. She said, "Yeah, I used to drink a lot during stress but now I have quit." Her test reports were telling her lifestyle. The liver was weak, enzymes were not working properly. Bilirubin, SGOT/SGPT was quite high, Haemoglobin and iron were low, cholesterol was beyond the range and vitamins were deficient too, but rich in Erythrocyte Sedimentation Rate (ESR). "In this age, how did you manage to ruin your health like this?" I asked in a very sarcastic way. Her test reports made me angry and I was feeling very bad for the youth who is sinking in bad influence or stressful life.

"Ma'am, mujhe pata hai ki Adamaya ki health achi nahe hai, but aap ke paas bohut umeed se aae hai. Doctors ki medicine bhi chal rahi hai par yahan aane ka reason iski sehat puri tarah theek karna hai. She is living far away from us, bachon ka kya hai bhukh lagi to kuch bhi kha liya bahar ka," her mother said in her defence.

I said, "The parameters can be controlled but what guarantee you are giving me that aap ki beti fir ye parameters pena hi pahunchegi? Stress will follow you everywhere, so will she drink alcohol like water?"

Adamaya looked at me with filled eyes and said in a heavy voice, "I will not do it again. I know that I was busy being so stupid that I did not take care of my health. Now I can understand what I have done to myself. Sometimes I shiver for alcohol but I didn't touch it from the last one month. Please help me to regain good health, abhi toh world tour par jaana hai mujhe, bade paise kamane hai, toh achi health bhi toh honi chahiye na." And then she had changed the entire aura of the cabin by her serious joke and a cold smile.

I asked her to give me 6 months to work on it, visit me on every 15th day and talk to my team on every 7th day. I planned more of detoxification for her liver and diet. To boost the formation of new RBCs, I added lemon, oranges, more salad, etc.

She followed all my instructions with some cheatings in between because she was a stress eater too. Her jaundice was treated in one month and the rest of the time, I gave her Immunity-boosting to increase iron and "tie the cholesterol in its range" kind of diet like spirulina, palak, garlic, etc.

I clearly remember my last meeting with Adamaya and her mother. Adamaya hugged me and said, "You have no idea what you have done for me. Aisa nahi hai that in this journey my motivation didn't break, but the only thing which kept me going was your first day anger about youth and stress. It was much needed for me because before that time, no one scolded me in that way. So thank you so much aur bus ab paise kama kr world tour par aish karungi,but without alcohol." She winked and laughed.

Take Away tip: Be high on life, not on anything else!

Forever High In Spirit, Yours Dietitian Shreya!

BEYOND MY BOUNDARIES

JAUNDICE

Mrs. Asha, 49 years

I had an appointment on call from Paonta Sahib. That was my first ever online case, so I was very excited about it too. I called, that was a landline number and a male took the call. I told him, Mrs. Asha took the appointment for today. He said, "Oh yes! I am her husband, Vinod. Can you just hold for a minute, I will call her to talk to you?" Our conversation started like this:

"Hello, ma'am… I am Asha; I have taken your appointment."
"Hi, Mrs. Asha. I am Shreya. How are you?"

"I am good, thank you."

"So, what is the concern? How may I help you with your health?"
"I have jaundice from the past 2 months."

"Okay, is there any history of it?"

"I had some issues in the past. It all started with an acidity attack. In the upper side of my stomach, I had severe pains. I visited the government hospital here for that, as it didn't get under control by medicines. They used to give injections of pantoprazole to me and I came back home. This was like a tradition for 3 months. The pain was severe and they kept on injecting me.

I have restricted myself from having excess tea, smoking, fried food and ghee. But it was all the same. Then my daughter came home and asked about this; she scolded us and asked us to go for a scan. We did go for a scan and got to know that I have gall stones. The gall bladder was full of stones. But that time, I was not able to take the call for surgery. So, I delayed it for some time.

But the pain came again and we visited a hospital in Dehradun for a checkup. They said my condition was not good. There is a severe infection in my liver because of obstruction in the bile duct. We were not prepared for it but I got admitted to the hospital. The titer of jaundice was high, the liver was inflamed too, and the pain was severe. In that condition, they didn't take the risk of surgery but treated my liver and controlled jaundice. So, I was in the hospital for 10 days.

After one month, my gall bladder was removed surgically. But my bilirubin is still not in a good range. Doctors told me that my liver is still a little inflamed. It might be due to the injections of pain killers and pantoprazole.

It's been 2 months of surgery but my bilirubin level is the same. My daughter told me about you and that you can help me with food which will control my inflamed liver."

"Okay… you have been through a lot of pain but this was due to your negligence. I wish you would've gone for the scan after the second attack of acidity or gall stone pain. But let bygones be bygones. We will focus on the future and I can give you a plan for your liver which will help you to control the bilirubin levels."

I planned more of carbohydrates and fats and avoided proteins in her diet. Her bilirubin level got controlled and inflammation of the liver was better than before. She was with me for 4 months and her liver was in good health at the end of the fourth month. Her family was really happy and her daughter met me to say thanks. When she visited, that was the moment I felt that I can go beyond my boundaries, beyond Chandigarh to help others.

When it comes to Health, there is No Defined Boundary for Dietitian Shreya

.

FATTY LIVER

Not So Required

The liver is the largest organ in the body. It helps in the digestion of food, store energy, and removal of toxins. When the liver is inflamed or stores fat around itself, it is called fatty liver. There are two types of fatty liver: Non-alcoholic and alcoholic fatty liver Disease.

Non-alcoholic fatty liver Disease: accumulation of fat in the liver while no drinking at all or drinking less of alcohol.

Alcoholic fatty liver is due to drinking alcohol in excess.

Fatty liver can cause fatigue, swelling in the abdominal region, pain in the upper right abdomen, enlarged spleen, enlarged blood vessels, etc. Obesity, Diabetes, age factor, food habits, intake of drugs, working of metabolism, etc. are a few factors which could be the reason for fatty liver.

Fatty liver is a silent Disease which will show symptoms when the problem reaches a higher level.

PIECE OF ADVICE

— High protein diet
— Less of carbohydrates and fats in the diet
— Avoid alcohol if you drink
— It's a condition that can be serious if you neglect it and can be easily reversed if you don't show negligence towards your health.

PUT HER FIRST

FATTY LIVER

Mansi, 24 years

When my video on the heart in 2018 got viral and people were approaching me for the same, I got an invitation for a health talk in the corporate sector on the same topic. In that health talk, I was very happy because the session was very interactive. It was not like one person speaking — they all were taking interest in the talk and asking so many questions.

There was a girl named Mansi, who was at the age of around 24 and was asking some very intelligent questions to me regarding heart Disease. I asked her if anyone at her home was having heart Disease? She said that her mother has high blood pressure and high cholesterol. I gave her many suggestions regarding the same and she was happy to know the answers.

After that, I said goodbye to the amazing time I had spent there.

The next day was the same in the clinic — people came to meet me for their good health and took advice from my side. There I was surprised to see Mansi with her mother in the clinic. The previous day, she took an appointment with one of my staff members when we were at their office.

She greeted me with respect and her mother was very kind and humble. Then I got to know that from where did Mansi get her traits of kindness. We were talking about her mother's health as she had told me about her health previously; I was all in to give her my best. Her mother told me that Mansi was also a patient of Diabetes who was taking medicines for it.

I told her to get some tests done regarding the same and likewise for her mother. When the reports came, her mother was quite healthier than Mansi. Her mother was having only one problem of high cholesterol but Mansi had Diabetes and fatty liver. I asked her why she was not taking care of herself? She said that she had been suffering from Diabetes from last year but did not have any idea regarding fatty liver.

"I don't drink; my lifestyle is not that bad, then why am I having fatty liver?"

I told her, "Fatty liver is not always because of alcohol, but also because your lifestyle is not correct. If you are taking too much stress, if your metabolism is slow, then your body is not healthy to convert your food into energy. It can be easily treated; don't you worry about that."

I started her mother's diet as well as that of Mansi. I suggested she take methi dana, Jamun Sirka, eggs, amaranth, more of salad was restricted in her diet plan and to have an adequate amount of water intake.

She said, "I am quite healthy so you don't need to work hard on me. I can handle my health easily but kindly concentrate on my mother's health."

I told Mansi, "Your health is not that good, so I cannot ignore your health and simultaneously, I am taking care of your mother's health also. I am spending my mind on both of you."

She started visiting the clinic every 15 days with her mother and this pattern followed for 3 months continuously. After that, when the tests were repeated, the level of HbA1c and fatty liver was better but could get controlled in another month.

Her mother's report had absolutely reversed and the doctor asked her to drop her medicine too. She took the diet further for one month and she was quite happy but she was happier for her mother. She was thanking me for her more.

That day I found out what the meaning of unconditional love of a daughter is.

Take Away Tip: Let the love expand, not the lever.

Dietitian Shreya!

ENTERTAINMENT IN LIFE

FATTY LIVER

Mrs. Manjot Kaur, 37 years

I was running a summer body challenge in my clinic. Many people enrolled themselves for that summer body challenge. That was for one month and the winner would get a family holiday package.

In my Amritsar clinic, Mrs. Manjot Kaur enrolled herself for the same challenge. She started the diet for her obesity, her weight was 98 kg in the starting when she was enrolled. In this kind of challenge, every person got the same kind of diet plan so that we could find out the winner. In that case, we didn't change the diet according to their requirement. And the same diet pattern was shared with Mrs. Manjot Kaur.

She was following it very dedicatedly but her weight loss was very less, so she visited the clinic and said this is not the kind of diet through which she can lose weight.

The diet counsellor over there told her that this was a challenge in which 50 more people had enrolled and it was already told that they can't change her diet. But yes, they could help her by giving her some suggestions. So she had started asking her about her daily routine and how she followed the diet the previous two weeks.

After speaking to her, she got to know that Mrs. Manjot Kaur was an alcoholic and would drink almost 5 times a week. She used to drink whiskey, wine, and beer or whatever she had. And after a physical examination, she found swelling in the abdominal region too. She asked Mrs. Manjot Kaur to have some tests done for her liver.

When she got the reports of her blood tests, she found that the range of her fatty liver was quite high. Her SGOT/SGPT levels were 57/80 and her sonography reports were also showing the same results. That was the reason she wasn't able to reduce her weight and also because of her high acidity problem.

She contacted me regarding this case because Manjot Kaur was enrolled for the challenge and she couldn't change her diet by herself so she contacted me and I took care of the case personally.

I spoke to Manjot Kaur on the phone when she visited the clinic in Amritsar. I told her about the health of her liver and the reason for her obesity. She needed to quit alcohol or reduce it so that we could treat her liver easily. Else it would lead to serious damages to her liver.

She told me, "It is very difficult for me to quit alcohol because this is not a habit developed over a day or two. I have been drinking for 5 years like this. I belong to a defence family. My husband is in the BSF and my son is in the NDA. I used to be alone at home and didn't have anything to do, so I started entertaining myself through a bit of drinking. I thought that it was a matter of time and kept enjoying that way. But after a long time, I got to know that I was facing some serious drinking issues."

I told her that I could totally understand her situation right now, but it was not healthy for her liver. How could she take something else to be more important than her health?

She said, "I am helpless in this but I will try my level best to quit it slowly."

I planned the diet according to her calorie intake because she took high calories with alcohol. I did not plan high carbohydrate and fats in her diet. Instead of that, I planned more of proteins like egg, amaranth, oats, barley, less of fruits and more of salad and I told her to avoid raw salad.

She started taking alcohol 4 days a week, then 3 days a week, and then came to one day a week.

When I went there to meet and greet, she came to meet me and said, "How different my life is! I don't need alcohol to entertain me anymore. Now I find relaxation in reading and yoga. I am into cooking again and feel happy after so long. The swelling in my abdomen is almost gone and my weight is 72 kgs now. I am really grateful to you for helping me and inspiring me to be me again"

Take Away Tip: Happiness needs no big reason, Celebrate every moment!

Happily Yours, Dietitian Shreya!

DIGESTION GERD & IBS

Before we start the story, let's understand the basics first!

The digestive system is set up of the gastrointestinal tract also called the digestive tract or GI tract. GI tract helps to digest food and give energy, growth, and cell repair to the body. If digestion doesn't work properly due to any reason, then it may cause GERD, indigestion, IBS, acidity, etc.

GERD – GASTROESOPHAGEAL REFLUX DISEASE

Stomach acid flows back into the mouth from a connecting tube called the esophagus. This acid irritates the lining of the tube and one can feel the burning sensation in their throat or that tube. GERD causes heartburn, severe acidity, indigestion, and coughing, vomiting and severe pain around the chest. Obesity or pregnancy is a common condition when one can be introduced with the problem. It's a big lifestyle Disease which can be due to alcohol, fried food, and lack of physical activity or exercise. Diagnosis of GERD includes- upper endoscopy, ambulatory acid probe test, esophageal manometer or with X-ray of the upper digestive system.

IBS- IRRITABLE BOWEL SYNDROME

IBS is a chronic Disorder of the large intestine. It is a cluster of intestinal symptoms which carries cramps and pain in the abdominal region, bloating, mucus in stool, diarrhoea, or constipation. It can be controlled by a good, healthy lifestyle and management of stress. Its symptoms could be weight loss, rectal bleeding,

vomiting, Anaemia, and Diarrhea, which helps in diagnosing the Disease.

PIECE OF ADVICE

- Find the root cause of your health issues. Sometimes we indulge ourselves too much in the symptom rather than the root cause.
- Digestion problem starts when we don't have enough fiber, water, physical activity or have an excess of fried and oily food, caffeine intake, and obesity.
- Keep a check on your belly fat because maximum health issues start from there only.

APPROPRIATE FUEL

GERD

Mrs. Amandeep, 46 years

I had a day out for myself after a long time and to spend it, I went to paint because that makes me happy. I went there and poured all my stress, thoughts, and tiredness out. I was happy that day because I got to meet many good artists; people were enjoying each and everything about that place. When I was about to come out, I came across a familiar face. I went to her and said, "Hey! Hi, Kiranjot; remember me? You came to the clinic last week with your mother, Mrs. Amandeep." She greeted me well and said, "Yes, of course. I do remember." "How is she now? Is she feeling good?" I asked further. "My mother was hospitalized last weekend. So, I just came to this place to divert my mind," she answered. I asked what happened to her.

"She had chest pain and a burning sensation; we thought it was a heart attack and we will lose her but luckily she is better now. It was a severe acidity attack and GERD. She was in severe pain at that time. I couldn't have imagined it; she was shrieking loudly. Doctors gave her injections and admitted her for 3 days; those days were horrific. The doctor said if this condition remains the same, then she will no longer be around us."

I was feeling so bad for her but when we were talking about her mother, I was remembering our first meeting. She told me about her mother's condition in front of her. But her mother was not in favour of taking any help from my side and was not even ready to take a diet plan for herself. I tried to convince her but she was there to meet me only because Kiranjot had forced her and asked her to meet me once. But after the counselling session, she left the clinic without letting us help her. I told Kiranjot on the very same day to take care of her. She is treading on this unhealthy path and will pay soon for this negligence. And a severe attack happened after that.

I asked her again, "Let me help your mother and I promise this condition will not happen again." She nodded and said she will bring her mother to the clinic tomorrow, positively.

The next day they came. Mrs. Amandeep said, "I will go on your way only for 1 month because my family wants it. I know you will not treat it, like doctors." I just smiled and started her diet plan in which I added jaun sattu, less of proteins, no raw food and less of fruits. The first two weeks of her diet guided me towards what was the real trigger for her so I avoided that stuff completely. And after a month, she said, "I am feeling much better now and I am not scared of the pain in my chest anymore. So, I want to continue further with my entire consent."

Within 3 months I treated her GERD, acidity, and its bad symptoms. But lifelong, she needs to take healthy food because our stomach is a body part, not a junkyard. We need to protect our bodies by giving an appropriate fuel to it.

Wish you a happy digestion always!

Yours Dietitian Shreya

BIG ENOUGH

IBS

Ruchi, 24 years

"Hi, Ma'am. I am Ruchi." "Hello, Ruchi. How are you?" "I am doing good."

This is how our conversation started on a shiny hot Sunday.

I asked her what she does and why she is visiting me alone? She said, "I am 24 years old and I am big enough to go anywhere alone." Then I saw her form and the column of age. She was not looking like a 24-year-old girl. I said, "Fair enough; just asked casually." "Of course, it's okay," she said.

"I live in Baddi and am working in a pharmaceuticals company as a mechanical engineer. My weight is a major concern for me and I thought let's give a try by getting nutrition properly. I live in PG (paying guest) there. So, it will be great if my diet plan will be prepared according to the menu."

I asked about her weight, was she thin like this always or any sudden change? She said she was like this always. Her present weight was 37 kgs only, after reducing 4 kgs during her job. "So, do you feel any other problem? Like constipation, loss of appetite or frequent loose stools?" Yes, I go to the washroom frequently, especially after having meals. Sometimes I feel nausea and loss of appetite. I eat a lot of junk food; in the evening, I have sandwiches, cold drinks, chips or samosa because, on the way back to PG, I feel hungry so I eat whatever I can."

I told her that she has IBS, according to the symptoms she had told me. "Yes, the doctor told me once about it. But I was too busy with my job so I didn't pay any attention to it," she added further. "Had you taken proper care of yourself, you would not have lost this much weight from your body. But it's okay, we can gain it back."

I started her diet according to her comfort level and tried to increase her appetite also. I planned almond milk, eggs, soup, fruits, salad, makhane, potato, jaggery, chicken soup, etc. which helped her gain her weight and reduce the symptoms of IBS too. When she had completed her journey and gained weight, she was looking like a 24-year-old girl. She was happy and her happiness made me happier.

Take Away Tip: A good eater is certainly a good man!

Eat Wisely. Dietitian Shreya!

OBESITY

Age Is Just A Number; The Weight Isn't

Obesity is a very common and underestimated condition, especially in India. Denial of this condition can cause some serious health issues. Obesity is a Disease on its own and also a hub of many Diseases.

In adipose tissues, unnecessary fat accumulation is called obesity. This accumulation can impair health. Obesity can be due to your genetic factors, laziness, over-eating or lifestyle. It can also be the symptom of other medical conditions like sleep disturbance, stress, PCOD, menopause, etc. When one gets overweight, some find it normal and feel comfortable in their skin but others feel a bad shape, consciousness, depression and low self-esteem due to their obesity.

All you beautiful people need to understand that being overweight or obesity is not a healthy condition. Small things lead to big things and if we take care of these small things, bigger things will take care of themselves on their own.

Obesity is defined by BMI i.e. BODY MASS INDEX.

BMI is a measure of the relative body fatness to evaluate risk factors associated with obesity. Our weight is categorized in different parts

Underweight — if BMI is less than 18.5 Non-Obese – 19-25 BMI Grade I — 25-30 BMI

Grade II — 30 – 40 BMI

Grade III — Above 40 BMI

PIECE OF ADVICE

- We like eating potatoes but we don't like to be one, so don't be a potato and move yourself
- Physical activity is important
- Healthy food is necessary
- Don't over react
- Have a good night sleep and stress-free life
- If you find your weight is increasing then do find the root cause of it and consult your Dietitian too.

BEING HEALTHY IS IN TREND

OBESITY

Dilraj, 32 years

It was evening and I was in a meeting with my team after announcing my pro bono cases and explaining how we will handle it from all over the place. Lakshman Ji knocked at the door and said there is a new walk-in appointment. I borrowed some time from the meeting and then asked Lakshman Ji to send her in.

When she entered the cabin, I kept looking at her. Her body language and fashion sense were very good. When she started talking, I was almost a fan of her. She said, "HI, Shreya. I am Dilraj, by the way, I like this green wall art on your back. It is really beautiful." I replied, "Hey, thank you so much but it is not as beautiful as you are. She wore such a beautiful saree with a halter blouse and wrapped it perfectly. I was admiring her for her style. I told her that she was looking very pretty and I loved her style and positive aura. She said that is why she was here.

She continued, "I am very fond of styles and I am a professor of fashion designing department at Panjab University, Chandigarh.

I am married and have 2 children. In 2017, I had my second baby through caesarian and gained weight after that. I was trying hard to get back into shape but it seems impossible sometimes. I love fashion and dresses. I want to be able to fit in my dresses again. I don't feel comfortable in a dress when my bulging skin comes out like this as an extra part of the body."

I told her that, She, need not worry about her weight, it can be controlled. Just keep your determination high. I found that she had Gestational Diabetes also during her second child so I had to focus on all over health, not only on the extra fat. I had given the plan with some heat-producing foods, protein, amaranth, jaun, more salad or fruits and advised her to have an adequate amount of water. Thereafter, every time she entered the clinic with a broad smile, glowing skin, lost inches, and weight. She was very happy to get her body back and got so many compliments for her beauty. I have suggested that she should model because she has that much capability.

I wish that Your wallet should be fat, not you.

Always helping you get in shape, Dietitian Shreya!

EDUCATION IS KEY

OBESITY GRADE 1

Mrs. Amrit, 43 years

We got a call from a lady Mrs. Amrit for a diet plan. She said, "I want to take a diet plan for weight loss as I am very obese and want to lose weight." My calling department asked about every parameter of her health but she said she had no problem and was a clean slate, just wanted to lose weight.

They had shifted the case to Chandigarh because Amrit lived in Mani Majra and wanted to take a diet plan from Chandigarh clinic only. The case was handled by Raman, my team member. Sunakshi asked her about her weight, height and medical condition if any. When Raman calculated her BMI, it was already in the obesity grade. She told everything to Mrs. Amrit but she didn't care about it much

and said, "In how many months will you help me lose my weight?" Raman said it will take time but it is not difficult.

Her determination was not good so her result was very slow. She was not used to measuring the progress on scale and inch tape. So Raman asked her to visit the clinic at once and if needed we could visit at your place, but she denied. Raman deciphered that probably she had some issues.

Every fifteen days, we conducted a meeting to discuss each case so that the results would be good and the work could be done with maximum efficiency. When Raman told me about the case of Mrs. Amrit, I spoke to her on the phone and asked her to visit the clinic. After so many calls, when she visited the clinic, we found the other side of her story.

She said, "I am depressed due to my marriage. My in-laws and husband are not supportive. I have three children and my mother-in-law doesn't love any one of them. They abuse us and torture us mentally. I wish I was also an educated person, at least, my children wouldn't suffer like this. Today I am here because of my children and my mother. They have motivated me to come here and talk to you directly. I am a stress eater, so whenever they do something to us, I eat a lot at that time. This is the problem that I am facing."

Her story was heart-melting but I found out how education is important for anyone. Education is not about having a degree; education is awareness about right and wrong. She shouldn't tolerate all this but she was unaware of the outer world, right and wrong, to stand for herself and her children.

I designed her diet according to her. She had a craving for paneer, eggs, spicy food, so I planned paneer salad in between, eggs, chamomile tea, lemon water, jaun, amaranth, raitas, and fruits. Told her to let sunlight enter the house, listen to music, indulge herself in some activity, and install fragrance diffuser in the room so that she wouldn't feel depressed anymore.

From then to the next five months, she didn't miss any meeting and was doing great. She is more like a free bird now because she got the confidence from her body. We have suggested her to join some kind of course too so that she can face this world with her head up.

No One Else Can Save you; But You Yourself

Yours Dietitian Shreya!

UNFORGETTABLE

OBESITY GRADE 3

Aayushi, 24 years

I got a WhatsApp message from my college friend that she is sending her friend's daughter today to me for weight loss. I told her, today will be tough but yeah, I will meet her tomorrow if it is okay?

She said it won't take time because she is in sector 35 only. I couldn't refuse her and after a long discussion, agreed to meet her.

When she entered the clinic, I was having my evening meal in the cabin. I asked Aarti, my office coordinator, to send her in because she is known to me. She entered the cabin and I offered her to sit on my black couch because I wasn't doing any formal meeting with her. I asked her about her bad health. Her weight was 158 kgs and BMI was 43.5 at the age of 24 years. It was a shock for me.

She told me that, "I was quite healthy in my school days but after entering college life, I was into a very bad company. I was having patch-ups and breakups, which made me a stress eater, unhygienic and almost a sloth bear. You are not the only one with whom I am consulting about my health. I have been to various Dietitians but I didn't feel that they were doing a good job. So, I kept on shifting and now I am here. I want weight loss before 25th September i.e. exactly after 4 months from now."

She told me everything by herself; I didn't need to ask any extra thing. I explained the science to her and how the body works. And said, "This weight loss result is not a one-way thing, you need to be very determined and focused on what you are aiming for."

She said she will do it; she just needs a diet plan. I started her diet plan. I restricted her junk food and food timings, sodium intake, intake of fats and excess sugar. After giving her a diet plan, I walked with her to the gate and she introduced me to her friend who was waiting for her in the waiting area. I said bye and wished her luck with the diet.

She visited the clinic every week but did not get the proper result that I was expecting. She lost only 2 kgs in one month, with 1 inch. When I asked her about diary and cheatings, she said she forgot the diary at home and did small cheatings but just on one day. After one month, she refused to take the diet further; when I asked the reason, she said you are not helping me in reducing my weight. I tried to convince her that she was not following the diet properly and had lots of cheating in between. But she didn't listen to me and did not take any diet.

I texted my friend: "Aayushi left the journey in between but she needs urgent help. Tell her parents to talk to her and convince her for the diet." "Okay, I will talk to them," she replied.

After almost one year, I was out with my family and friends for a day trip to Kasauli. We were sitting in a café there and having fun. I noticed a boy staring at me. He looked familiar to me but I didn't recognize him and thus ignored. When we were about to leave the place, he came to me and said, "Hello, ma'am, how are you?" I said "Sorry. I don't recognize you." He said, he came to my clinic one year ago with Aayushi.

Then I could recall her and said, "Oh yes! How are you? And, how is she?" He said with watery eyes, "Aayushi is not alive now. We were getting engaged on 25th September and she wanted to look perfect on that special occasion. Her lack of determination of healthy eating led her to surgery.

Doctors cut down all the extra fat from her body and asked her to take care of herself but she was not good at it. She was an unhygienic person and got infections. Infections got severe and she died because of that. I wish I could have helped her at that time and could been a support to her; at least she would have survived."

After knowing that, I didn't utter a word and left the place. From Kasauli to Chandigarh, I didn't say anything and didn't cry too. I felt completely blank and couldn't think of anything. I have made a policy of putting undetermined people in a category of special care so that this will not happen again with anyone.

Hunger for Love is much more concerning than for food!

Always in an effort to feed you right, Dietitian Shreya!

CELIAC

Not a Big Deal

INTRODUCTION

It is a chronic inflammatory Disorder due to gluten intolerance in the small intestine. The person is known to be allergic to gluten dietary products. It is an autoimmune Disorder generated against gluten in atopic individuals. In celiac, mucosal surface impairs and leads to failure of absorption of nutrients. Undiagnosed celiac Disease in children might have severe consequences. Gluten is the most common ingredient in human nutrition (composed of proclaims and glutelin).

Everybody does not show the same symptoms in this condition. Some show the problem of indigestion and show the deficiency in the body after intake of gluten.

Type 1- normal intraepithelial lymphocytes count

Type 2- presenting aberrant intra-epithelial lymphocytes.

CONDITIONS ASSOCIATED WITH CELIAC

- Diarrhea
- Constipation
- Abdominal pain
- Anemia
- Enteropathy
- Ulcerative Jejunoileitis (extensive ulceration of the intestinal mucosa)
- Osteoporosis
- Down syndrome
- Turner syndrome

- Neurological Disorder
- Increase the risk of Type I- Diabetes
- Increase the risk of Thyroid

REASONS

- Genetically transferred
- Environmental factors
- Viral infection

DIAGNOSIS

- Check the presence of genes encoding for MHC class II proteins including human leukocyte antigen HLA-DQ2 and HLA-DQ8.
- Anti tissue transglutaminase antibodies
- Anti – gliadin antibodies
- Deamidated gliadin peptides
- In vitro gluten challenge test

PIECE OF ADVICE

- Cut down gluten from your diet for life
- Even mustard seeds are rich in gluten. So, if you are purchasing anything from the store, try to have at the label. It always mentions if the product is gluten free.
- Check on your Vitamin B12
- Gluten is not a friendly protein
- Shaurya is not celiac but still, he is having a gluten-free diet from his childhood and his body strength is more than a year-old kid.
- It's a "blessing in disguise".

SHINING LIKE SUNSHINE

CELIAC

Harkirat, 14 years

Gurkirat Singh was one obedient and nice client of ours. He was waiting for his meeting in the waiting area. There is a TV screen in the waiting area, on which my videos run. He was watching a video of gluten-free overnight oats recipe.

Aarti asked him to go to the cabin for the meeting. When he entered the cabin, I greeted him like I always do in Punjabi 'Sat Sri Akal Sardar Ji, kive ne tussi?' And we both laughed aloud. He was not comfortable in any other language than Punjabi. He replied, "Sat Sri Akal madam Ji, assi vadiya han tussi dasso." And our conversation started. I was asking about his migraine and knee pain but he was somewhere else in his thoughts. I didn't interrupt him and waited for him to come back. He said, "Oh sorry! Kuch keh re c tussi… mera dhyan kisi hor hi val c…" (Sorry! What did you just say… was thinking about something else)? "Ki hoya tuhanu?" (What are you thinking?) I asked in a very fun way.

"O tussi kuch dassreh c oss video ch jo bahar play kiti hui c… ki c oho?" (You mentioned something in that video which was playing in the waiting area. What was that about?) "Which video?" I was confused. I rang the bell of the reception area and my Team mate came in. I asked her, which video was playing outside. She told me that it was a recipe video of gluten-free overnight oats. "Haan ohi gluten… ki Honda ae ehe? Meri bhtiji nu v koi dikkt ae edda di kuch." (Yes… gluten. What it is? My niece is facing some gluten-related problem too). I got to know that there is some serious problem so

I asked him some more questions about her. "Oh 14 saalan di ne hje, tehje ton hi ohnu eh gluten ton dikkt ae. Sannu smjh hi ne aunda ki kriye asi. Menu v pichle hfte hi dseya ohna ne," (She is just 14 years old and at this small age, she has some problem with this gluten. We really don't know what to do. Even I got to know about it last week only) he replied.

After listening to him, I asked him to bring her here along for a meeting. He agreed and she accompanied him the very next day. Her face was red and there were rashes on her arms. And being a teenager, she was irritated with all the skin problems and the medicines she had to take.

"Hi Harkirat, how are you? Wow! What pretty eyes you have. You look like your mother more than your father, right?" I talked but she just smiled and blew the conversation. I asked her mother about her medical condition and test reports. Her mother showed her reports to me in which the IgE levels were very high and in food allergy test, she was allergic to many food products like wheat, almonds, nuts, cotton dust, etc. When I saw her dietary recall, I was not at all shocked because many people don't know what to take or what to avoid in this situation. I wanted to talk to Harkirat but she was not interested because I was just another person or doctor for her with whom she was meeting and would get no result, according to her.

I didn't force her to talk to me and started the diet plan by sharing all the dos and don'ts in those allergic conditions. I did not plan anything for her with anything she was allergic to. I planned more of gluten-free oats, amaranth, ragi, rice and avoided wheat, bread, rye, all kind of dry fruits and advised her to use mask whenever she went out. I made my instructions very clear to her mother so that Harkirat would not face any discomfort anymore. I said all the very best to Harkirat but in reply, she said, "At least you didn't give me the drugs," and left the cabin with a smile.

She followed the dos and don'ts properly and on the 15th day of our meeting, she met me with a big beautiful smile on her face and greeted me well. Her face was much better than before and rashes on the arms were a bit less. She said with a broad smile, "I did follow the instructions and I am feeling good after a long time. I am not ashamed to go to school anymore. This time, the other students were not behaving strangely with me after they saw my face, thank you, ma'am. "I smiled and said, "I am meeting you for the first time, the last time who came to see me was a child with irritation but now you are shining like sunshine. Stay positive and trust me." And the journey continues...

A life without hope is like a fish without water

Hoping for your never-ending happiness, Dietitian Shreya!

A VIDEO CALL

CELIAC

Jyoti, 8 years

Meena Ji is an important part of my personal life. For a very long time, she lent a helping hand in taking care of my two munchkins and she is like family to us. One day we were all sitting together at around 9 am when Meena Ji got a call that her daughter had met with an accident and was admitted to PGI. She was in a lot of tension and left in a hurry. I was thinking of meeting her daughter too. In the afternoon, I left for PGI from the clinic to meet her. When I reached there, I got to know that she was in the trauma center of PGI. They don't allow visitors there, but I called Meena Ji out, gave her some money and food to eat.

A visit to PGI was very painful for me as I saw a huge number of patients sitting or lying outside. I also witnessed a lot of patients who were in a lot of pain lying on the statures. On the very same day, I announced to do pro bono cases (free of charge diet plans to those who couldn't afford it) in every clinic. Many people from my team went to different hospitals to do such a noble deed. As a result, I reached to a child named Jyoti (8 years old), who was suffering from gluten intolerance. She lived in Mandi Gobindgarh with her mother and two brothers. She had lost her father in a road accident and her mother was poor and couldn't afford any expenditure. My team from Patiala got their address from the government hospital. The doctor told, "Jyoti is suffering from gluten intolerance and her body is too skinny now, the stomach remains upset, the energy level is very low and she is Anaemic too. I have given her the treatment for Diarrhea, Anaemia, low energy but they are not taking care of her gluten-free food. This time I have seen rashes on her body, though the rashes were small, it was an indication of elevation in the allergic reactions. If you can help them, then you will save the life of a child."

My team went there and met them. These were the special therapeutic pro bono cases that were only handled by me. My team asked every small question to her mother like what was she giving her to eat? What items were included in it? What problems Jyoti was facing? How better she was? What supplements was she giving to her? By that conversation, they came to know that she was still having gluten in her food and was not even taking the supplements which were given by the doctor. They called me to discuss the case and told me everything that they had written in the form for Jyoti. I switched the audio call to video call (thanks to digital India). When I saw her for the very first time, I was thunderstruck. She was very skinny and looked malnourished and her mother was the same; she was thin and all were living in a small room. As I was talking to Jyoti, I found that she was scared to talk to me. I made her comfortable but she didn't talk much. I talked to her mother, she had tears in her eyes and said, "Mennu ne pta, tussi sadde tk kive pahunche ho. Pr sche badshah tuhanu trkkiyan deve, te tuhanu te tuhade parivar nu achi sehat deve. Tussi sade lae jo karre ho ohde lae dhanwad." (I don't know how you people reached us but God will bless you with all the success and good health. Whatever you are doing for us, it's commendable and thank you for this.)

My eyes were full of tears but they didn't come out. I just thanked God for this life and started her diet with the "No Gluten" agenda. The next day my team again visited there and gave them gluten- free food stuff like eggs, quinoa, amaranth, ragi, jowar, gluten-free oats, and rice, with vegetables, fruits, and her supplements, which the doctor had written for her. They gave them a list of "things to avoid", written in Punjabi (Wheat, barley, rye, wheat germ, graham flour, and semolina). They gave a diet to her mother also so that she could live a healthy life.

My team had to visit there in 15 days because they did not have any phone to communicate. When my team member went there, he found the room locked and asked the neighbours. They told him that they had left for Moga with their mama (mother's brother). Their mother had died 10 days ago.

While coming back from the factory, a car hit her and she died. So, her brother took all her kids to his native place.

When I got to know about it, I sat quietly in my room and I could feel that pain of losing someone very close to the heart. Till today, I am not able to forget Jyoti. I wish, in the future, she will try to contact us again and I just want to meet her once.

Body can die, energies can never

Spiritually Yours, Dietitian Shreya!

BONES

Strong As Always

INTRODUCTION

Bone is a growing tissue that is made up of collagen (a protein for flexibility of bone) and calcium phosphate (a mineral for bone strengthening). Throughout life, bones change in size, shape, and position and also once in a lifetime, old bone is removed and new bone is added to the skeleton. The common problem which can be faced by a woman is Osteoporosis.

OSTEOPOROSIS – In Osteoporosis, bone loss begins either due to the breakdown of bones or decreased levels of bone formation. When bone mass lessens, it leads to structural abnormalities making the skeleton fragile. The composition of minerals, porosity of bone, and the presence of micro-fractures are all important in determining bone strength. Genes, lack of nutrition, and bad lifestyle are also responsible for bone weakness. The process of Osteoporosis accelerates in a woman during the time of menopause.

CAUSES

- Genetic abnormality
- Nutritional deficiency
- Muscle weakness
- Hormonal Disorder
- Increasing age
- Use of the excess of glucocorticoids
- Inflammation in the body
- Lack of exercise

- Immobilization
- Smoking can also have negative effects on bone mass and strength.
- Misalignment

DIAGNOSIS

- Joint pain with activity
- Transient stiffness in the morning or after rest
- Reduced range of motion
- Bone swelling
- Radiography and dual-energy X-ray absorptiometry (DEXA) bone scan

PIECE OF ADVICE

- Lifestyle modification
- Fall prevention
- Consider the fragile fracture
- Gluten-free diets
- Soaked and peeled Almonds
- Jaunsattu as a calcium supplement
- Have calcium citrate, not calcium carbonate if you are taking a calcium supplement
- Do not have Calcium Citrate of 1000mg at one go, should divide into two, 500mg each.
- Leafy vegetable kale, sesame, ragi, pinni, alsi, makhane
- Bamboo Silica tea
- Amino collagen
- Eggs

- Wheat has a component called phytic acid. It causes the malabsorption of vitamins, calcium, and iron if you want your bones to be healthy.
- Milk is not the only source of calcium. It has an acidic pH which buffers out the calcium from the bones.

SUGAR IN CHAI WITH MATHI

OSTEOPOROSIS

Mrs. Shashi, 61 years

One of my mother's sisters, Mrs. Shashi, visited our house for several days. Genie, my mother, and she used to talk a lot in the evening while snacking. She walked less or you can say she avoided it.

Genie asked her, "You walk very less and whenever you walk, your speed is very slow. Is your health okay?" She told her that she was having severe knee pain and the DEXA scan showed severe damage to her bones. Her daily routine was badly affected by this knee pain. Sometimes she woke up in the middle of the night due to this pain and took pain killers. She was putting on a lot of weight after this knee pain started. She spent her day with her grandkids and ran behind them but now it was too difficult for her. Day-by-day her family noticed that she had started finding it difficult to walk up to the kitchen also.

Maasi is a retired bank employee and had spent a well independent life but this old age was bringing new challenges to her. The doctor suggested her to go for knee replacement surgery. I told her that even if she decides to get her knees replaced, she needs to maintain her weight as too much weight can affect the knees again.

Her son and daughter-in-law were not in favour of the surgery, as they also agreed with a lack of nutrition in her food. Maasi loved consuming mathi with her sugar filled chai (tea), and her usual breakfast used to be vada pav most of the time. It was very clear to me that she was not consuming anything specific for her bone health.

During the discussion with her, she told me that during her menopause she gained at least 8 kgs and then never reduced it. Probably, that was the only reason for this situation. As jaun sattu has more calcium than milk, it was planned in her diet. I suggested her to consume pearl powder daily, her vitamin D3 levels were also on the lower side, so eggs were an important meal and 15 minutes of sunlight exposure a day was an important morning routine for her.

As she sticks to the planned diet, her knee surgery was postponed for the next 7.5 years. She reduced her weight as well as increased her bone strength. And these years were comfortable and painless for her. I am happy that I could gift her effortless days.

Take Away Tip: A tree with a weak root will fall

Dietitian Shreya!

PAMPER THE INNER HEALTH

OSTEOPOROSIS

Mrs. Jaya Thakur, 38 years

Three years back I went for a workshop at a private bank. I met Mrs. Jaya Thakur. It was a 4-day workshop and I noticed that most of the people entered the office around 10 a.m. and left by 7 p.m. They never got proper time to see the sunlight and there is barely any physical activity. Mrs. Jaya was serving her last year in the bank and was about to get retired. During our first session, I built a good connection with her but soon I noticed that she was finding it difficult to walk.

On the third day of the workshop, I noticed that she wasn't there at the session. I thought it might be her off that day. On the fourth day, I woke up in the morning and got my daughter ready for school and had my all-time nutritious breakfast — Egg bhurji with oats roti. On my way to the bank for the last session, I kept a small gift for Mrs. Jaya, but when I reached there, she wasn't there at her desk. After the session I asked my team to call her; Mr. Mukesh, her husband, answered the call and informed that she had twisted her feet in the washroom and when people at the hospital got her DEXA scan done (a test for bone density), they found her to be in the initial stage of Osteoporosis.

I sent good wishes to her via message and requested her to visit the clinic once she felt better. After two weeks I met her at my clinic, she was worried about her bone health and said, "Shreya, I am very scared, I've become so fragile that I can fall anywhere and will get some bone broken."

I replied, "You don't need to be scared, I am here and can get you out of this."

But internally I knew it will be a slow and steady process, this was something you can't change overnight and in case of a female after deliveries / pregnancy, post-menopause you lose so much from your body, it requires a lot of care and nutrition to pamper your inner health. It was a medical challenge to treat her Osteoporosis but I would never give up on this. The personalized diet designed for her had makhana, broccoli soup, ragi, pearl powder, pearl millets, kasha, and most importantly, eggs.

Our hard work paid off and her DEXA scan showed 12% betterment. Anyone who finds themselves in such a situation, I would say you shouldn't despair. A good diet and determination can improve the situation for you.

Don't let the spirits die

Enthusiastic To Give You The Right Diets, Dietitian Shreya!

CANCER

Undesired Multiplication

INTRODUCTION

Cancer is the uncontrolled division of cells in the tissues or organs. Uncontrolled division of cells can be triggered by different carcinogens or when the body's normal function disrupts. In women, there are three Cancers which are prominent i.e. breast Cancer, cervical Cancer, and ovarian Cancer.

BREAST CANCER

When breast cells grow uncontrollably, it forms breast Cancer. It can be benign or malignant and can grow in different parts of the breast simultaneously. Every year, 1 woman out of 10 is diagnosed with breast Cancer. Breast Cancer is asymptomatic in the early stages. Breast pain is an unusual symptom that happens 5% of the time.

RISK FACTORS

- Age
- Family history of Cancer
- Personal history of breast Cancer or any lump in the breast
- Artificial hormone intake
- Damage of DNA
- Genetic mutation
- Exposure to estrogen

SIGNS AND SYMPTOMS

- Hard skin
- Breast lump
- Change in the size of breast and nipple
- Nipple discharge
- Lymph node changes
- Breast or nipple pain
- Redness
- Swelling or inflammation

DIAGNOSIS

- Screening - mammography
- Biopsy

TREATMENT

- Surgery
- Chemotherapy
- Radiotherapy
- Hormonal therapy
- Targeted therapy

CERVICAL CANCER

Cervix is the lowest part of the uterus. It connects the uterus with the vagina. Usually, cervical Cancer is very slow-growing, but in certain cases, overgrowth of cells of the cervix can invade the other tissues. Cervical Cancer is the 2nd most common cause of Cancer death in developing nations.

SIGNS AND SYMPTOMS

- Frequent blood spots or bleeding
- Heavy and longer periods with a foul smell
- Bleeding during and after intercourse
- Increased vaginal discharge
- Bleeding after menopause
- Unexplained and persistent pain in the pelvic region / or back
- Pain during urination
- Blood in urine and stools

RISK FACTORS

- Infection with a virus called HPV human papillomavirus
- Sexually transmitted infection
- Smoking

DIAGNOSIS

- Pap smear test
- Annual screening
- Colposcopy
- Biopsy

OVARIAN CANCER

Cancer begins in the ovaries (part of the female reproductive system) that produce eggs as well as estrogen and progesterone (female hormones). There are two ovaries, one on each side of the uterus.

Generally, ovarian Cancer remains hidden until it has spread within the other areas like the pelvis and the abdomen. At this late stage, ovarian Cancer is more complicated to treat and can be lethal.

RISK FACTORS

- Old age
- Inherited gene mutation
- Family history of ovarian Cancer
- Estrogen hormone
- During menarche or menopause
- Obesity
- Lack of nutrition
- Lacking in physical activity

SIGNS AND SYMPTOMS

- Bloating or abdominal swelling
- Quickly feeling full when eating
- Weight loss
- Uneasiness in the pelvic region
- Changes in bowel habits, such as constipation
- Frequent urination

DIAGNOSIS

- Blood tests
- Imaging
- Pelvic exam

PIECE OF ADVICE

- Frequent screening of breast after the age of 30
- Consult your doctor if you find any abnormal changes in the body

- Maintain your weight because underweight, overweight, or obesity can hamper Immunity
- Work on your Immunity otherwise chances of recurrence of Cancer will be there
- To increase Immunity, have spirulina, eggs
- Avoid raw things, it can cause infection

IT'S ALL INSIDE

BREAST CANCER

Mrs. Harminder Kaur, 57 years

My calling department had fixed an appointment for me from Bathinda; a lady named Harminder Kaur, her age was 57 years. She verified each and everything about me regarding my work, clinics around India and the success rate. My calling team told her everything about the success rate and all the cases we have seen in our career. She was in Bathinda and she had so many clinics around her but she decided to meet me directly with her case (which was serious).

She started her journey early in the morning so that she could arrive on time at the clinic to meet me. She had visited with her son, Gurpal Singh, along with her reports; she was suffering from breast Cancer. Adding to it she told me that she had a small lump in her breast and the doctor told her that it was probably not an issue but she should go for mammography and a few tests for confirmation.

After mammography, the doctor told her to go for biopsy also because they had some doubts about the lump and in case that lump is Cancerous then they would need to operate it and if it is not a Cancerous lump, then they will treat it differently. She was done with her biopsy and the doctor suggested lumpectomy.

She was worried about the surgery because she had a phobia of hospitals and the surgical instruments after the death of her husband. He met with an accident and died in the hospital during a surgical procedure; so, she avoided being to hospitals ever since.

But the lumpectomy was important so she had to undergo it. After surgery, the doctor started therapies i.e. radiotherapy and chemotherapy. When she came to me, doctors had suggested her 12 chemotherapies and she was already done with one chemotherapy.

She told me, "It has been a lot and I can't handle it anymore; it is like death to me or perhaps death is easier. I can't live life in this hope that probably one day, I will be better or one day I will not feel like this anymore. After my husband, I have my children and their families to live for and I know may be my life is not that precious but I don't want to die right now because I am happy with my life, whatever it is showing me. The most awful thing for me is that I am losing my hair in this procedure."

She was crying in front of me because her hair was losing its strength and there was heavy breakage. She further said, "My husband loved my hair and we are Sikhs and for us, our hair is our pride. I know maybe you find me to be a crazy woman who is thinking about her hair and dying but if anyone else was in my shoes, then they might have understood me."

"You have already passed the most difficult time of your life like losing your husband, decision of lumpectomy and chemotherapy. So don't let your hair come in between your treatment," I requested humbly.

I further said, "Yes, the chemotherapy has some effects on your body, hair, energy, and Immunity. After the chemotherapy, you will feel dizzy, nauseous, sleepy and low in energy; but it will help you to live a Cancer-free life.

You need to gather your strength now and push your treatment towards betterment. If you already took the step then don't be afraid of swimming in the middle of the ocean. You have already crossed half of the ocean, now it's halfway to cross. It's up to you, how will you cross it: happily, or sadly.

I can help you to get through this positively but that inner strength you need to find in yourself. One can always show you the path to you by showing the path but you are the only one who can walk on it."

Her Immunity was low and she was emotionally weak too; so, I talked to her son about most of the things because she was not in the state to listen. Her son also told me about how shattered they were when they got to know about his mother's Cancer because he already lost his father and now, he did not want to lose his mother so he was here to get some help.

Her doctor suggested him to go to a Dietitian; especially, during this period because she needed healthy food during her chemotherapy. The doctor told them my name for this case. I heard the family very carefully and found out how people feel when they find out something like this about their family members. I started the diet with boosting her Immunity and diet which could provide more energy to her. I told her to avoid raw stuff like raw salad, raw fruits. I provided eggs, spirulina, moringa tea to her so that her Immunity could boost up. I told her to have barley roti with light vegetable soups, boiled eggs, etc.

I told her to take the second opinion on the chemotherapies because twelve chemotherapies are more than enough. When she came the very first time, I found her a broken lady but now after 4 months, she is much better by health and her mind.

She said, "It was difficult for me to get over my bald head but it is a phase of life and it will cross like any other phase of life. Now I am strong enough to handle it.

I know it was important for you to make me healthy but yes, you were right, that one can show me the path but only I could make it possible to cross it. I felt nauseated, weak after every chemotherapy of mine. I felt like, why it is happening to me only? But after that, the one thing I got to know is that if a situation is happening in your life, then you need to be patient and that situation will pass.

Thank you, Shreya, for the help. If you were not there for me and you were not helping me through this journey of chemotherapy, then probably I would have not crossed this phase like this."

Wishing you A very Happy Sunshine Forever!

Brightly Yours, Dietitian Shreya!

DON'T BE AFRAID

CERVICAL CANCER

Mitali, 20 years

I still remember the day I first met Mitali. Walking into my cabin, she had a concerned look on her face. I asked her straightaway that what was it that had her so worried. Narrating her story she said, "I first found urination painful, almost a year ago. It was frequent. I was terrified to go to the washroom because it was very painful. I told my mother about this, she said that probably it's a urinary tract infection (UTI). So, we visited a doctor. He said, "It's okay. At this age, children go to public toilets and sometimes, a bit of unhygienic lifestyle affects as her age is 19 years." I was not an unhygienic person but yeah, I used public toilets because, at that time, I used to stay outside the house more.

He gave me the medicine and it was all cured after some days of taking those medicines. But after some time, I started to face the same problem again and it was more painful than before. The doctor gave me the same treatment as he gave the last time and told me to follow some precautions to avoid this kind of problem in the future.

I followed his instructions and took the medicines again. I got treated but my vaginal discharge increased. In the beginning, I didn't take it seriously but after that, it elevated. I did not tell my mother because if I told her, she would have taken me to the doctor again and he would have repeated the procedure as he did before.

After a few months, after painful urination and vaginal discharge, I passed blood through urine and I felt persistent pain in my pelvic region. After the fifth day of my pain, I told my mother about all these things which I had been going through for the last 3 months.

Blood in the urine happened for the very first time but the rest of the symptoms were the same: that persistent pain in the pelvic region, pain during urination, and heavy vaginal discharge.

When she took me to the doctor, he prescribed some tests for me which were highly recommended at that time. These tests included ultrasound, Pap smear test and CA 125. The doctor told my mother about these tests, not to me" Mitali described her situation to me.

"I was badly shattered at that time," her mother continued. "I felt a sharp pain in my chest — that pain was of fear. Fear of, if the tests showed up with a positive result? What if the matter will be serious? What will happen to her life? How much pain will she face further? My mind was full of questions. Her age was just 19.

I called Hiten, her father, and told him about the situation, 'She is our daughter, I can't dare to face Mitali and tell her about the tests, please come home soon. 'Hiten and I were in the living room and prepared ourselves with positive thoughts that we will tell her about the tests because the doctor said that there is a possibility of cervical Cancer. We told her about the tests in the morning before we left for the test lab and she didn't say anything after that, she didn't react, and she just shut herself."

Mitali said, "When the reports came, I was like my life is over. I was in the early stage of Cancer. Probably, I was not afraid of the treatment but I was afraid of not living the life I could live. I didn't tell my parents how precious they are to me, I didn't talk to my elder sister properly till now, I am not living my life the way I dreamt. The doctor asked me to start the treatment so that we can control the damage. I have been suffering from the past 5 months with the problem and now I want to end it. So, I agreed to take the painful procedure."

"Her surgery is done and the process of chemotherapy is on", only a few are left. She felt dizzy, did vomit, felt pain in the body and mood swings. I don't want to see her like this anymore. I was very patient through all this time but now my patience is over and now I am just a helpless mother of a fighter daughter.

We have heard about your cases of Cancer, one of my colleagues suggested us to come here because you helped him in the case of his wife with breast Cancer."

I heard both of them and I felt, I was there in every moment of theirs and could feel the same pain. My eyes filled with tears like them, I hugged both of them and told them how strong they are and now I will be another family member who will help theirs fight this battle.

I gave her diet like moringa and spirulina for her Immunity, jaun, blanched vegetables, more of protein and steamed salad. She is still here with me in my healthy family and we are on it.

These kinds of cases are always neglected because of unawareness regarding the issues of the reproductive system.

Go and see your doctor if you feel anything abnormal in your body.

Dietitian Shreya!

TAKE STAND FOR YOURSELF

OVARIAN CANCER

Ripple, 36 years

For ovarian Cancer, I have a name that suddenly pops up in my head, the name is Ripple Kaur. She had given a testimonial for me regarding her recovery from ovarian Cancer without any surgery, radiotherapy or chemotherapy but with the help of diet only.

I still remember the day when she met me for the very first time with her Mother. Both of them were very nice to me and they were very good persons. Ripple had some serious health issues. She was facing a problem with her periods and was detected with ovarian Cancer because her Cancer Antigen (CA) was 125.

She was obese, nutrition was not proper, and physical activity was not a part of her life. Ripple told me that she had spent her whole life around her family, husband, and children. And she didn't care about her health properly so the result was that she was facing lots of health issues in her life. She was not able to wear any kind of footwear because her feet were swollen.

She told me, "I am not able to walk properly because of the pain in the body and especially in my feet. Pain in the body, facial hair, uneasiness and swelling around my pelvic region brought me to the doctor. He recommended certain tests like pelvic examination, hormonal study, Pap smear, and CA 125.

When the doctor examined my body and test reports, he got to know that my Cancer antigen was quite high i.e. 125 which made me feel like I am stuck in the middle of a fire and didn't have any idea about the next step if it will gift me my life or burn me.

My head was banging with questions like, what will happen to my kids and my family for whom I have spent my whole life. My mother started crying in front of the doctor and told him: She is my only child and I will also die if she will face anything like that. I don't have any issue with the money but I want my daughter to get treated and be healthy."

When they entered the clinic, I found that she had multiple problems in her health and if she was not treated for all these issues, then probably she would die but I was very positive and told her that her CA 125 can be controlled easily but only if she took care of herself properly.

We started her diet with high protein, less of carbohydrates and fats, no raw food was recommended to her, she needed to blanch or steam everything like salad or fruits or vegetables.

She was getting her checkup done after every 2 months and in every report of hers, I found that her CA 125 was getting controlled. Her CA125 came at 35.2 from 125 and that was a huge achievement for them. I have learned from her that we women spend our whole life around our family, for husband and kids but we always neglect ourselves in between so I want to tell you to take a stand for yourself.

A strong will means half the battle won against Cancer! Keep the will to live high!

Yours Rock Solid, Dietitian Shreya!

KIDNEY

Not Just A Bean

The kidney is the filtration system of the body. It filters blood and excretes waste products from the body in the form of urine. Kidney Diseases start when it doesn't work properly. It is due to high blood sugar levels, high blood pressure, not get enough blood, etc. Water retention in the body that leads to swelling in the limbs, shortening of breath, abnormal urine output, etc. are some early symptoms of kidney Diseases.

Chronic kidney Disease (CKD) is a gradual loss of kidney function; fluids, electrolytes and body wastes built up in the body. Kidney failure is the end stage of CKD, which is lethal without dialysis (artificial filtering) or a kidney transplant. In CKD nausea, vomiting, muscle cramps, swelling in limbs, shortness of breath, high blood pressure, fluctuation of blood sugar levels are the symptoms.

PIECE OF ADVICE

— More of barley is recommended
— No raw food
— Water intake should be under the supervision of your doctor
— Light vegetables should be taken
— Less of sodium and potassium intake

A NEW PHASE OF LIFE

CHRONIC KIDNEY DISORDER

Shweta, 23 years

Shweta's Bua, Mrs. Pooja Kohli, used to visit the clinic for weight loss. I was astonished to see her as I was meeting her after a year now and she was looking quite maintained. This time a new enrollment, Shweta was visiting with her. She told me, "She is my niece and she is diagnosed with Critical Kidney Disorder. Our world has turned upside down."

I turned to Shweta and started asking about the symptoms. She said, "Initially, I started feeling tired and weak but kept ignoring these symptoms as I thought it was the result of skipping meals. As all these symptoms were getting worse and I noticed this foul smell and foamy urine, I told my mother and she took me to a doctor. After an initial examination at the hospital, I was referred to nephrologists and was admitted to the hospital for another 5 days. I don't remember how many times they pierced through my veins, already I was in pain and that hospital smell was slowly killing me."

The experience narrated by Shweta was horrible and she had just entered a new phase of her life and with it, she entered in big trouble too. She said, "When I got to know about CKD the very first time, I thought nothing could be worse than this. I took a week to deal with the situation and after talking to my loved ones, I decided to keep my spirits high and since then, I have never given up on my life. I have decided to live every moment of life." This nature of Shweta was very uplifting for her family also.

Mrs. Pooja Kohli said, "Ma'am, she is good at managing her emotional state but I can rely only upon you for her physical well-being."

I assured them that I will be giving more than 100% for a soul like Shweta, it's not every day that you get to meet people like her.

I studied her reports thoroughly. As her uric acid and potassium levels were high, we were supposed to eliminate all the calcium-oxalate food from her diet starting from palak-paneer to excess of caffeine. Her water intake was restricted to 2 litres a day by the doctors and majorly, barley was planned in her diet.

She is leading a life with better health now but the battle continues for her. She is a perfect example of liveliness and strength.

Life is beautiful even without the Filter

Originally Yours Dietitian Shreya!

SIBLINGS

CHRONIC KIDNEY DISORDER

Priyanka, 32 years

It was Raksha Bandhan and we ran an offer on our social media for all the brothers-sisters. Atul took an appointment for his sister through my Instagram account. She had started her boutique recently and started noticing a swelling around her ankle. She thought it was because of her hectic schedule and a new profession, so didn't bother to go for any check-up.

Then she started feeling dizzy progressively and was losing weight rapidly. Finally, she decided to get her general check-up done as the swelling was increasing day-by-day. Along with this, she started getting fluctuations in her blood pressure levels also. When she received her medical reports, she was diagnosed to be Anaemic and couldn't believe her renal function test, so she got it done from another laboratory, but unfortunately, it was the same.

Atul was all teary-eyed. He said, "During this auspicious day, all the sisters pray for long lives of their brothers, but today I want to wish her a long and healthy life."

I told Atul, "The journey won't be easy for her as she has to endure a very strict diet where low protein, low sodium, low potassium diet would be recommended to her. She has to cut down on refined sugar, coffee, and bakery. This means she needs to be on low potassium vegetables and has to blanch them every time. The grains are also supposed to be restricted." He was ready to reach every possible limit for his dear sister. It was a challenge for me also; as her diet had to be high in calorie but low in proteins but Ms. Priyanka was very supportive, she wasn't a fussy eater and I could focus on better results with her.

Atul never missed even a single meeting along with his sister and now it's been more than 4 years, she is leading a healthy life without dialysis. Her renal function tests, uric acid, GFR, and electrolytes showed a great improvement and it's under control.

I wish them a lifelong bond of love as they have already been sharing from their childhood.

Yours Dietitian Shreya!

POLYCYSTIC OVARIAN DISEASE

A Trend

Polycystic ovarian Disease (PCOD) is a hormonal Disorder causing distended ovaries with tiny cysts on outer edges. It is because of genetic factors, poor lifestyle, obesity, Anaemia, and other environmental factors. PCOD symptoms consist of irregular or no menstrual periods with severe pain, unwanted facial hair, acne, and pigmentation on the face, pelvic ache and trouble in conceiving, alteration in mood, depression, irrational behaviour, and obstructive sleep. It can be diagnosed by ultrasound, blood tests, and hormonal study.

PIECE OF ADVICE

- Avoid having dairy products, especially milk
- Say no to fried food and gluten products
- Control on weight is priority
- Increase heat-producing food
- Maximum protein and less carbohydrate and fats
- Good night sleep and physical activity are equally important
- Avoid gym so that testosterone level is in the range
- Be happy even if it's tough

EMOTIONS ALLOVER

PCOD

Mrs. Payal Garg, 26 years

It was a busy day at the clinic as it was Valentine's Day. We were having 52 appointments and my husband was also coming to pick me up. On the very same day, Mrs. Payal Garg, a lookalike of Bollywood star, Bipasha Basu had fixed her appointment in the late afternoon hours. She visited the clinic with her parents, and before I could say something, she said that she came to know about us from a friend and got good reviews from her but still couldn't believe that PCOD can be treated.

On this, my answer was simple, "PCOD is directly linked to your weight gain. If you gain even a single kilogram, your tendency to form a cyst will increase and it is like a vicious cycle which makes you gain more weight."

Mrs. Payal said, "I have never got my regular periods after the delivery of my second kid and I am in pain most of the time. I am also facing severe mood swings and because of this, my husband has also started ignoring me. You can notice this skin pigmentation, facial hair growth; somewhere I have lost my identity."

She had lost her confidence and even started ignoring public gatherings. Initially, when I checked her reports, her ultrasound showed that she was having multiple cysts along with disturbed prolactin levels in the hormonal study. I could imagine her situation and the discomfort she had to undergo every month. Though I had already treated an uncountable number of hormonal imbalance and PCOD cases, this was unique in terms of Payal's emotions.

True happiness knocked at our door exactly after 6 months. I was so excited that we decided to go live on my social media and make this big announcement. Payal was so emotional that day, she couldn't control her tears even in front of the camera. I grabbed her hands tightly and her smile and tears of happiness were my trophies.

In her diet plan, I kept gluten-free food to work on her hormonal imbalance / PCOD and included mostly fiber and zinc for prolactin specifically. Milk and high sodium were a big no for her diet. Keeping her hydrated was a major task while getting water retention removed from the body. To cleanse her body, I made sure she consumed enough anti-oxidants and Vitamin C in the form of lemons.

Now she dresses up like a diva and as is my profession, I love bringing happiness to everyone.

Beauty lies in the eyes of the beholder!

Helping you stay beautiful always

An Empath, Shreya!

HOPE OF HAPPINESS

PCOD

Pallavi, 20 years

Now I am going to tell you about a beautiful experience I had at my Panchkula clinic. Pallavi was diagnosed with PCOD at the age of 20 and her gynaecologist told that it could bring some complications in conceiving or during pregnancy but at that time, she had no idea about how was this important to her. She ignored and kept living her life.

She was focused on her career and other important engagements, and then it was the time when she had to move into the next phase of her life when she got married to Abhishek. After a year of their marriage, they decided for conception, but even after trying for months, the couple wasn't able to conceive. After trying for another one month, the couple had good news but this didn't stay for long as Pallavi had a miscarriage after 6 weeks.

This was not all for her; all the relatives started poking her for this. After so much of bullying, she built up a suicidal tendency.

Luckily, Abhishek was very cooperative and he constantly tried to keep her happy.

When she visited the clinic, I wanted to give her all possible results, so we made a plan where I needed to work on her egg quality, along with her muscular weight. I checked out her egg quality reports, it was 16mm but was supposed to be 20 mm. Her diet had maca root powder, eggs and maximum of proteins. She was highly allergic to citrus so she had to cut down on tomatoes, lemon, and apple cider vinegar. I also had to work on her Immunity so that she was completely ready for conception.

After 5 months, her entire family visited with a big box of dark chocolates and now the couple is blessed with a baby boy.

Destiny is Pre-Planned, Wait for an action!

Yours compassionate, Dietitian Shreya!

ENDOMETRIOSIS

All About Thick and Thin

INTRODUCTION

Endometriosis takes place when the lining of the uterus (endometrial) develops outside of the uterus or on other pelvic organs, such as the ovaries or fallopian tubes. Endometrial tissues coagulate and bleed outside the uterus, just as the normal endometrial does during the menstrual cycle inside the uterus. Due to this outgrowth of lining, women can face painful sex, cramping during intercourse, painful urination or infertility. It may appear due to genetic factors. Endometriosis can also occur as a result of direct transplantation—in the abdominal wall after a cesarean section, for example.

It can spread to:

- The ovaries
- The fallopian tubes
- Ligaments that support the uterus (uterosacral ligaments)
- The outer surface of the uterus
- The lining of the pelvic cavity

PIECE OF ADVICE

- Say no to dairy products, fried food, and gluten products
- Check up on your weight scale and inches
- Good night sleep and physical activity are equally important
- Avoid gym

80/20 CALCULATION

ENDOMETRIOSIS

Shiney, 28 years

Shiney was a bright student and after completing her schooling from Ahmadabad, she cracked the entrance exam and got admission in IIT Mumbai. But this was not all for her. She wanted to reach higher heights and she had the caliber for the same. On one beautiful day, all her dreams came true as she got selected for a project at MIT, Massachusetts, US. Her parents had no limits to their happiness and they were showing the letter to every possible human on Earth.

She got another mail from MIT, in which they had mentioned about female fitness. They had sent a picture of a female and asked her to be like that; however, Shiney was overweight. I still have that picture in mind

— it was a picture of some lean and tall model.

The challenge began from there. Shiney had endometriosis and it was a task to lose those 5 kgs within a given period and we had to build her muscles. As she was working out vigorously in the gym, she noticed some changes in her body. She was working out hard; she was getting broad shoulders and wasn't losing as much weight with the workout. So, I explained the science to her that 80% is what you eat and 20% is your physical activity, so she needed to be more particular with whatever she was putting in her stomach.

Here, we began to fulfil her ambitions by defeating thickened endometriosis. We worked on two simple rules –high protein, high fiber. I tried giving her less fructose, more fiber in the form of salads and cut down gluten from her food completely. Feel-good hormone inducing foods were also planned for her to work on her mood blues and together we aimed for it.

Now she has moved to the U.S. and was doing muscle-building diet there with isometric open environment work-outs and no one is happier than me for her biggest inspiring story.

Take Away Tip: Vulnerable or Resilient? The Choice is Yours!

Eternally Yours, Dietitian Shreya!

OPTIMISM IS THERE

ENDOMETRIOSIS

Mrs. Pratibha, 33 years

Mr. Rohit and Mrs. Pratibha were from Gujarat who visited my clinic in Chandigarh. They had watched a video of my YouTube "Why am I not losing weight?" and booked their appointment from there. They were enough to pay me a visit from so far but during their counselling, I was introduced to a sad reality.

Pratibha said, "I am a Hindi professor in a college and Rohit is a manager in State Bank of India. During our late 20s, we were completely focusing on financial stability but as we both are now in the 30s, we want to extend our family. I had been a very healthy person; I used to participate in every activity of my college, I am particular about my walk, I am maintaining a healthy weight. But I had never thought that someday I will be facing these kinds of issues to conceive."

The couple consulted a doctor and she was diagnosed with Endometriosis. They had heard this word for the first time. She never had any pelvic pains, irregular periods or any of the symptoms. The couple thought maybe this is because they had entered their 30s and that these are the common issues. So, they kept waiting for natural conception, but due to this ignorance, she hit early menopause and all of their hopes shattered. She was facing mood swings and pain in the body after menopause. She had shown symptoms of depression too. Now she is 42 and they don't have a kid.

But still, the beautiful couple has been optimistic about life, and here we are on a page to start working on their good health.

I wrote this story so that it can be a lesson for women around to at least get an annual regular check- up of their fertile health. It is not only about having children but it can save you from many upcoming health hazards also.

A request to all the women to please do not ignore the signs, symptoms of your body and have a regular checkup after you turn 40!

Yours Womaniya!

FIBROIDS

Growth is Not Always Welcome

INTRODUCTION

Fibroids are generally present in uterus known as uterine fibroids. They are non-Cancerous growth and aren't related to any risk of uterine Cancer. It can be single or multiple and distort the shape of the uterus. Fibroids can cause heavy and prolonged menstrual bleeding, pain in the pelvic region, frequent and painful urination, constipation, backache or leg pains. Heavy bleeding can cause severe Anaemia. It can predominantly occur during the time of menopause; it runs in the family history also. It can be diagnosed by transvaginal ultrasound, MRI and hysteroscopy.

PIECE OF ADVICE

— Dairy products, especially milk is a big no
— Control your weight
— Increase heat-producing food
— Maximum protein

I AM A WOMAN

FIBROIDS

Anu, 28 years

I was known to Anu as she was a relative from my in-laws. Anu and Akshay had a beautiful dream wedding in Rajasthan and we enjoyed to the fullest there. Everyone was saying she had got a kingdom and was blessed to have a family like that. People blessed the couple and after enjoying the wedding, everyone went back to their respective places.

I got a call from Anu after 2 years of their wedding. I sensed this awkward sadness in her voice as my husband handed over the call to me. Before I could ask her, she started sobbing and said, "Bhabhi, I have been diagnosed with uterine fibroid as we were planning to conceive from the past one year. I have lost all hopes and I can see a harsh change in my family's behaviour. I am not responsible for what's happening to me. What is my mistake that I am a woman and have to produce kids?"

As a clinical nutritionist, I knew what to do; I didn't want to sympathize with her with words only but wanted to help her out with conception. Unfortunately, I can't change the society and the way it has burdened females with different taboos.

When I started working with Anu, her diet was completely off milk and excess of sodium. As she used to have excessive bleeding, she was also diagnosed to be Anaemic. So, I planned jeera + coriander water in her diet and we reduced 6 kgs of weight. As she lost inches from her stomach, they conceived and now her daughter has started going to school.

I am glad that her in-laws are also good with her now.

A lady can be defeated by only herself. No one else!

Strongly Yours, Dietitian Shreya!

HOLIDAYS

FIBROIDS

Mrs. Anjali, 35 years

Mrs. Anjali came to the clinic for joining a weight loss regime. When I checked her form, she was having symptoms of hormonal imbalance i.e. hair fall, mood swings, acne, and facial hair growth. Apart from these symptoms, she had severe pain in her abdomen region. So, I asked her to see a gynaecologist and take a consultation for hormonal study and ultrasound.

As a clinical nutritionist, I needed to work on every aspect of Anjali's health but as she wasn't having any medical reports so we had to stick to weight loss journey. Her husband was posted in the army and she was waiting for him to come home for his holiday as she wanted to take him along for the doctor's consultation. We were doing amazing with the weight loss and she used to ring bells every week and those high-fives shared all the positive vibes between us. The only worry we had was that she wasn't losing as many inches from her abdomen region. It was that time of the year when her husband was about to visit her and it took almost two months for getting her complete reports. It was at this point that we got her ultrasound report that she had a uterine fibroid of the size of a 4-month fetus.

This time she visited the clinic after skipping the meetings for 20 days. She went for a small break to Mussoorie with her husband and when she came back, she had excessive bleeding during her periods. It was so bad that she wasn't able to leave the house for any other work.

My counselling room was filled with silence as the doctor's recommendation for uterus removal was lying in front of me. Her husband was really worried for her because in the forthcoming week, he had to depart for his duty and they had no other option than getting her operated.

We could have saved her from the surgery if we acted on time and took it seriously as even a single day causes a toll on your health.

I wrote this story so that while sipping on your favourite cup of tea or while enjoying a daily soap on TV, don't ignore your body's call.

Get a proper diagnosis and lead a better lifestyle.

Your Diet-Mate Forever, Shreya!

MENOPAUSE

A Much Required Pause

Menopause is a natural biological process that starts at the age of 40-50 years in woman. It is the time of the ending of the menstruation cycle. This menopause brings the relaxation time as there is no more need to use sanitary napkins but it also brings hot flashes, disturbed sleep, mood swings and bad temper, painful sex, depression, and weight gain. In this phase, a woman's body deals with many changes including variation in hormones and weakening of bones. It can be natural or triggered by any surgical removal of an organ from the pelvic region. Post-menopausal women are susceptible to Osteoporosis and heart Diseases.

Complications associated

- Heart Disease
- Osteoporosis
- Urinary incontinence
- Sexual function
- Weight gain at this time

PIECE OF ADVICE

- Eat healthily
- Take calcium to keep bones strong
- Supplement of evening primrose oil
- Steaming chamomile tea with ashwagandha
- It's very natural to gain weight and become grumpy after menopause. Don't worry, we are here and all you need is a tight warm hug.

OWE ONE

MENOPAUSE

Mrs. Harpreet Kaur, 45 years

I met Mrs. Harpreet Kaur at my brother's party, he is a DSP and Mrs. Harpreet is his colleague. I have been in touch with her from her training days. She has a pleasing and happy to go personality but this time, at the party, she looked anxious and stressed out.

I crossed the small staircase and went to her, gave her a tight hug to her and asked, "Is everything okay, aunty? You look tired. I have always seen you calm and happy, but this time your body is looking so fragile."

She said, "I have started getting hot flushes and am not even able to focus on my work due to mood swings and am having this severe body pain. Sometimes I am not able to explain my situation to people. I am losing confidence by gaining weight and due to this, my blood pressure is also shooting up. Recently, during our annual body check-up, I got to know that my cholesterol is also on the higher side, though I am not consuming any oil now."

I was worried about Harpreet aunty as she was a big support during my teenage years. There was this incident when a group of males were eve-teasing my friends, she proved to be huge support back then. Now it was time to return the favour, so I started working on her health.

A few tips from her diet are:

For high cholesterol, you not only need to eliminate excess oils but also an excess of carbohydrates. Instead of having fructose-rich fruits, I suggested her to stick to salads and to consume chopped garlic cloves empty stomach with water. For her high blood pressure, we eliminated excess of sodium from her diet, no namkeen, pickle, or papad were allowed and started with Ashwagandha at least once a day.

Evening primrose oil helps a lot in such cases, so we suggested her to consume it to avoid mood swings.

With all these tips, we delayed her menopause for another 3 years and now she has finished this stage and is living a happy retired life with her family.

Menopause is not just a pause, it is a new beginning

Yours Forever, Dietitian Shreya!

FEEL GOOD

MENOPAUSE

Mrs. Diljit Kaur, 50 years

It was a slow rainy day in Chandigarh and I was engaged in preparations for celebrating Ganesh Chaturthi at my clinic and home. I love Indian festivities and specifically, this time of the year is so emotional for me. Bringing Ganesh Ji home with a Dholi, taking care of Ganpati Bappa every moment, making Bhog and making him sleep after a long day makes me feel so pious and cleansed out mentally.

A special client, Mrs. Diljit Kaur visited the clinic. Why special? Because I haven't met a joyous lady like Diljit before. She has lived every single moment of her life. From her family to her friends, everyone has been a fan of her nature.

When she visited my clinic, she had achieved the stage of menopause and started with the after effects. Her knees had started hurting already, she gained 12 kgs of weight and was suffering from hot flashes and anxiety. As we needed to work on her hormones, stress, and weight, we started with correcting her lifestyle and meals. It had to be high in proteins and feel-good hormones, so chamomile tea was a major part of her diet.

I used to give her oats roti kneaded with mooli and onions for keeping it rich in proteins. Her favourite meal was moong dal with jaun roti, and for strengthening her bones, Ragi sheera was planned in her meals.

The right kind of meal and lifestyle helped her to lead a life with balanced hormones, managed weight, and a much energetic routine.

Life is easy, we just need to mind the bumps ahead!

Your Navigator, Dietitian Shreya!

MY INSPIRATIONS

"Namaste, Ma'am, I am Rajesh and she is my wife Pooja." A couple entered my office. I greeted them nicely and sat on the seat.

"Have you reversed Diabetes ever?" Pooja asked. I said with a smile, "Of course, it is possible."

"Aapne kabh ikiya hai kisi ko sahi? Nahi,matlab, maine suna hai ke Diabetes thik nahi hoti or agar pehle kam hoti bhi hai to fir se hojati hai," (Have you done this before? I have heard, it is not possible to reverse it or if it gets reversed, it will reoccur) she continued. I asked the concern of the couple first because they were terrified of something and the question arrived from that.

Mr. Rajesh told me with tears in his eyes that their son has been diagnosed with Type I Diabetes. "He is only 10 years old and 8 months back, his body was out of energy and his weight was continuously shedding in grams. We were taking it normally because, at this age, weight is not stable. Then we got complaints from his school and tuition that his performance in academics and sports was turning downwards. We scolded him badly for the poor performance but couldn't find the root cause of it.

We were trying hard to make him best in everything because he is our only child. Even after doing all that, the situation was not under control. He was very much irritated with us for whatever we told him to do. We thought he was just being a child with a lot of stubbornness.

On his holiday, we planned to go to his Nani Ji's place. When we went there, they asked us what happened to Naman; he looked very lean and pale. Is everything okay? Even we noticed the same but we had neglected it, but they asked us so many times, so we considered it. When we were in the sitting area of the garden, Naman came to us in anger and tears and we asked him, what happened? He said his cousins were not letting him play with them and when we asked them about it, they said that in a game of 60 minutes, he was running to the washroom every 20 minutes and due to this, their game was getting interrupted and they were not being able to enjoy it.

On the way back to Panchkula, we were talking to him and asked him why he is not doing well in studies and is he drinking too much water? He said, he studies hard but is not able to memorize things properly and the frequent urination was something which he did not notice. While we were driving, he said he wanted to go to the washroom again though 20 minutes before he had gone to the washroom. I said, "Just sit tight for some time, I will stop at the next filling station," but he said, "It's uncontrollable." He peed in the car and there was a foul smell.

When we changed his clothes, I noticed that his legs had only bones and no flesh. It was horrible to see our son like that. I could feel that fear, my heart was beating with the speed of a horse and my mind was shouting aloud of some terror. We took him to the doctor and he recommended some tests. We have done all his tests and he is Type I diabetic. The doctor told us that he is suffering from juvenile Diabetes as his mother is also Type I diabetic.

When the doctor told us about this, our world shook. The pain of insulin shots is intolerable for a kid and now he will have to experience it. That thought broke us both and we wished, that it was a bad dream and wanted someone to wake us up from that. But that was a reality, a horrible reality which we had to face. A reality we were not ready for.

We denied administering him insulin shots and wanted to try some other way to treat our child. But his condition was getting worse and we were not able to find any other thing except insulin.

Yesterday, we took the appointment of the doctor to take insulin shots but we saw your newspaper advertisement and took a chance to come here for him. He is not on insulin but his condition is not good. Please help us."

They were both crying like a kid, they were the parents who could do anything for their son. After this conversation, they called their son to the clinic; he was very thin and pale just as they had told me. I started talking to him and held his parents' hands together and told them that we would reverse his Diabetes.

I have started not only Naman's diet plan but also his mother's. We have more protein in the diet, eggs, jaun, methi dana, jamun sirka, kachnar's vegetable, kalonji, soups for NFeroza and for Mrs. Pooja, we have planned light vegetables, with jaun roti, jaun daliya, eggs, soups, methi dana.

They were with us for four months and when I received their reports in my hand again, that moment was cherishing. His HbA1c was less than 7 and C-peptide was within the normal range. The insulin shots of his mother had been reduced by the doctor. And Naman is still not taking any medicine or insulin for his elevated level of blood sugar. I remember the smile on his face and the progress in his health which inspired me.

When I shared Naman's story in my event on World's Diabetes Day on November 14, 2019, I got another case same as Naman but the only difference was that the girl was on insulin.

After the event, we met so many people: women, men, old age groups and kids who were dealing with Diabetes. There I met Palak, a cute little girl. When she entered the cabin, she wore a smile on her face and came with her parents. They told me that they had heard about Naman in the event. So, they were here for their daughter Palak. I met her and asked her a few questions, but when I saw her age on the form, I was a little shocked. Her age was 13years and her growth was like a 9-year-old kid. They told me that when she was 10 years old, her sugar level elevated. Her fasting sugar was 289 and random was 400. When she was admitted to the hospital due to a high blood sugar level, her doctor injected insulin into her and commanded them to give this insulin shot to her four times a day. They did not even ask them and just told them about insulin. From that time, she had been taking insulin shots. When I saw her reports, I was amazed by the doctor's deed. Her HbA1c was 7 and C- peptide was normal. Her body does not need any insulin shots. Her growth was stuck; she was not growing physically and mentally. She was under-confident when she was talking to me. She was not able to attend school because she felt shaky and drowsy. Her insulin was too much. I recommended she take a second opinion from the doctor and start the diet for Diabetes, energy, growth (mentally and physically), Immunity and muscles. She still comes to me and her insulin is reduced.

These kinds of cases are a true inspiration for me. Whenever I think that I have worked enough and need rest for some time, kids like Naman and Palak inspire me and tell me that there is a long way to go…

MY HEAD BANG MOMENT

On world Diabetes day i.e. November 14, 2019, we announced a free one-month diet plan for all diabetic patients, which could open doors for those who couldn't afford a Dietitian. And that announcement brought Sneha to us. On Sunday, November 17, 2019, Sneha, her father, and her mother came to the clinic. They met my team members Sunakshi and Rayshita first. Sneha was very thin, brown haired, fair and shy. She did not talk much when her counselling was going on.

Her father told, "For a very long time, she was not feeling well and her weight was losing continuously, which was our main concern. But people told us that it is normal at this age as she is a growing child; so we didn't bother much.

After some days, her body pain started and she felt very weak. When we visited the doctor, they gave us tablets for calcium and vitamin D3. They told us that this is just a deficiency and nothing else. We gave her the supplements but her condition was the same. She was not able to go to school due to dizziness. She was always sleepy and her frequency of urination increased. Doctors suggested some tests and they gave us iron supplements. But at the end of October 2019, when she was not able to walk properly and her weight reduced a lot, we had to admit her in PGI. Doctors did all the tests including HbA1c and her HbA1c was 13.6 on the 5th of November and fasting sugar was above 300.

Doctors told us about the situation and our life completely shook. We couldn't understand the situation but the thing we understood was she was not well. We asked doctors to control the sugar level and save our daughter. They gave her insulin shots to control the sugar level. Her C-peptide was 0.4 and the doctor told her to continue the insulin shot in her daily routine. We were very disheartened but to keep her well, we had to start the insulin shots.

From October end till now she is on leave from school too, so that she can take her meals properly. But from the very next week, she has to attend school so we are concerned about it. I got to know about your clinic from the local newspaper where the Diabetes event was mentioned. We are here if you can help us and our daughter."

Sunakshi calmed them down and asked them to show every report to her and took some time from them to discuss the reports with me. She called me and told me the whole situation, our hopes were less because her C-peptide was 0.4, but we decided to give our best for Sneha. I told Sunakshi regarding her diet and asked them to visit the clinic on Saturday.

We planned an open diet for her like eggs, chicken soup, barley, vegetables, chana soup, methi dana powder, and jamun sirka. Her mother told Sunakshi that Sneha's father is not having neither his meals nor his sleep properly, and has been crying since then. Sunakshi told them that they have to be strong for Sneha as this behaviour will make her weak not strong. They started like that and today on December 11, 2019, I have no way to show my emotions for God's grace. We have repeated all the tests to know how her body is responding to the diet. Just in one month, she dropped a few insulin units, HbA1c reached 7.4 and C-peptide is on 0.7. When I saw the reports of her C-peptide, I was crying like a kid with a big smile. It was not less than a miracle to all of us. Throughout their journey of just one month, Sunakshi and I were completely determined towards her and here was the result. Our journey is still in the middle of the ocean but now we are more positive and happier. Hence, this shows the Law Of Attraction and power of hope.

Highlights; HbA1c = 13.6 to 7.4 and C-peptide = 0.4 to 0.7 in 1 month.

THIS IS JUST THE BEGINNING

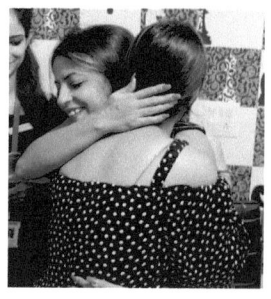

I might be ending this book but this is just the beginning of this never-ending topic of "health of women." I have connected with thousands of women and I got to know that they need to know themselves and the importance of their health. Whether it's Sarah, Aasha, Mridula, a mother, a daughter or me, we don't deserve bad health, depression, Diabetes or Osteoporosis. We deserve to be healthy and happy. My aim in writing this book is to reach maximum people and tell them to open a window of self-love, happiness, and health. If your health is at its peak, no one can pull you back in your life because you will be psychologically or physiologically healthy. Bad thoughts will never conquer you; you will never rely on anyone to do your stuff. These are the best feelings when you are no longer depending on anyone for your happiness and actions.

I have seen such cases when people lost their hope and said that they didn't want to take medicines, didn't want to go through surgery and asked, why they were a bedridden person, why they cry all the time or why they have these allergic reactions on their skin which makes them conscious. When someone in front of you says such things, you feel helpless and sometimes, to raise a ray of hope within them is the most difficult part of the treatment.

But my experience taught me that nothing is impossible. Don't give up on yourself or your loved ones, everything will be good and beautiful again. Good, healthy, and hygienic food, proper sleep, a bit of exercise and your hobbies can keep you alive, happy, calm, and healthy.

I am a strong believer in the law of attraction, so I know if you want something from the depth of your heart, you will definitely get it. Your hope, thoughts, and words are going to the universe which will make things happen according to your deep-down will. Think positive, take good nutrition, bring healthy thoughts and let the universe do its job of making your thoughts come to reality. Everything is interconnected and you should start from the core of the connection i.e. healthy eating.

As I said, this is the beginning of this topic, not the ending. So, I am here to help you and your loved ones. I am hoping you will share this piece of advice with maximum people so that the one who needs me, I can reach them. We can discuss it further and you can join me on my Facebook or Instagram page through my name 'Dietitian Shreya' and you are free to ask questions.

ACKNOWLEDGEMENTS

Life has been nothing less than a roller coaster ride for me. In this journey, some people were always there for me, held my hand and pushed me to do the best and stay positive in every situation. Whatever I am today and I have achieved would not have been possible without my papa, Mr. Arun Kumar Goel. He is my biggest inspiration towards being a good human, to help others and spread unconditional love. He is not with me today but I know, somewhere from heaven, he must be smiling and sending love to me.

Mrs. Asha Aggarwal, my mother, my genie has always been my rock. Her limitless love and care for me and my children shows the real strength of a woman. She is my mentor, who made me think about every small thing and taught me how to make my path. One can get success in the world when he/she is loved at home.

15 years of partnership through thick and thin, Ups and Downs has been commendable with my lovable husband, Sukhpreet Singh. He is a true partner, a wonderful person, and a perfect guide. Thank you for your guidance and help to make this book come true from my imagination. I couldn't have accomplished A Complete Diet Guide for Women in a lifetime without an extremely talented team.

I would not have been able to function successfully in this world as a daughter, mother, wife, and working woman without my team.

My special thanks to my women and my clients, who inspired me to write my experience in these pages and kept me going on the right path. Whenever I found myself tired of doing my job, my munchkins helped me to start with a sparkle again, playing with Saadgi and Shaurya gave me a good come back to the work field. Thanks for the generosity everyone; it gives me motivation to be ready to lend a hand.

www.ingramcontent.com/pod-product-compliance
Ingram Content Group UK Ltd.
Pitfield, Milton Keynes, MK11 3LW, UK
UKHW042001230426
12048UKWH00009B/476